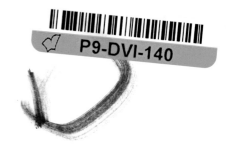

P9-DVI-140

DIABETESRISKS
FROM PRESCRIPTION & NONPRESCRIPTION
DRUGS Mechanisms and Approaches to Risk Reduction

Sam Dagogo-Jack, MD

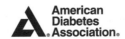
American
Diabetes
Association.

Director, Book Publishing, Abe Ogden; *Managing Editor*, Rebekah Renshaw; *Acquisitions Editor*, Victor Van Beuren; *Production Manager and Composition*, Melissa Sprott; *Cover Design*, Lawrence Marie, Inc.; *Printer*, United Graphics, LLC.

Printed in the United States of America
1 3 5 7 9 10 8 6 4 2

The suggestions and information contained in this publication are generally consistent with the *Standards of Medical Care in Diabetes* and other policies of the American Diabetes Association, but they do not represent the policy or position of the Association or any of its boards or committees. Reasonable steps have been taken to ensure the accuracy of the information presented. However, the American Diabetes Association cannot ensure the safety or efficacy of any product or service described in this publication. Individuals are advised to consult a physician or other appropriate health care professional before undertaking any diet or exercise program or taking any medication referred to in this publication. Professionals must use and apply their own professional judgment, experience, and training and should not rely solely on the information contained in this publication before prescribing any diet, exercise, or medication. The American Diabetes Association—its officers, directors, employees, volunteers, and members—assumes no responsibility or liability for personal or other injury, loss, or damage that may result from the suggestions or information in this publication.

Jane Chiang, MD, conducted the internal review of this book to ensure that it meets American Diabetes Association guidelines.

∞ The paper in this publication meets the requirements of the ANSI Standard Z39.48-1992 (permanence of paper).

American Diabetes Association titles may be purchased for business or promotional use or for special sales. To purchase more than 50 copies of this book at a discount, or for custom editions of this book with your logo, contact the American Diabetes Association at the address below or at booksales@diabetes.org.

American Diabetes Association
1701 North Beauregard Street
Alexandria, Virginia 22311

DOI: 10.2337/9781580406192

Library of Congress Cataloging-in-Publication Data

Names: Dagogo-Jack, Sam, 1954- , author. | American Diabetes Association, issuing body.
Title: Diabetes risks from prescription and non-prescription drugs: mechanisms and approaches to risk reduction / Sam Dagogo-Jack.
Description: Alexandria : American Diabetes Association, [2016] | Includes bibliographical references and index.
Identifiers: LCCN 2015030720 | ISBN 9781580406192 (alk. paper)
Subjects: | MESH: Diabetes Mellitus--etiology. | Prediabetic State. | Drug-Related Side Effects and Adverse Reactions. | Risk Assessment--methods. | Risk Factors.
Classification: LCC RC660 | NLM WK 810 | DDC 616.4/62061--dc23
LC record available at http://lccn.loc.gov/2015030720

Dedication

This treatise on the expected and unexpected effects of commonly used prescription and nonprescription drugs on glucose metabolism is dedicated to the medicinal chemists, physicians, and scientists who serve society by discovering and testing medicinal products for the alleviation of human suffering and to the research volunteers and test subjects who make such knowledge possible.

Disclosures

Dr. Dagogo-Jack is a principal investigator or coinvestigator for clinical trials contracts between the University of Tennessee and AstraZeneca, Novo Nordisk, and Boehringer-Ingelheim and has served as a consultant and an advisory board member for Merck, Novo Nordisk, Boehringer-Ingelheim, Eli Lilly, GlaxoSmithKline, Sanofi, and Janssen Pharmaceuticals. He also has served as an expert for Sidley Austin, and Adam and Reese, on diabetes-related litigation.

Table of Contents

Preface

More than 29 million Americans currently have diabetes and approximately 86 million have prediabetes. People with diabetes often also require medications for several comorbid conditions (including hypertension, dyslipidemia, depression, heart disease, pain syndromes). A vast literature abounds, however, on the potential adverse effects of numerous medications on glucose metabolism. There is, thus, genuine clinical concern that certain medications used for treatment of comorbid conditions and other indications (such as hormone replacement, contraception, infections) might worsen glycemic control in diabetic patients or trigger diabetes in others. These concerns influence therapeutic decisions in a manner that sometimes emphasizes avoidance of possible dysglycemia over effective control of the comorbid conditions. The same concerns may also weigh against the otherwise appropriate use of necessary medications.

The purpose of this concise book is to provide clinicians with actionable knowledge regarding the effects of various medications on glucose regulation and diabetes risk. Beginning with a brief overview of diabetes pathophysiology, the different drugs have been organized by class, and the scientific evidence for the diabetes risk and possible mechanisms have been presented for each drug. The agents discussed include widely prescribed medication classes: antibiotics, antidepressants, antihypertensives, bronchodilators, sex hormones (androgens, estrogens, and oral contraceptives), glucocorticoids, lipid-lowering agents, nonsteroidal anti-inflammatory drugs, acetaminophen, and thyroid hormone. Although less widely prescribed than the foregoing list, atypical antipsychotics, HIV antiretrovirals, immunomodulatory agents used in transplant medicine, gonadotropin-releasing hormone analogs, and human growth hormone also have been included because of the interest generated by their link to diabetes risk. In addition to medications used in ambulatory practice, this work includes a discussion of total parenteral nutrition (TPN)–induced hyperglycemia, which is associated with increased morbidity and mortality among hospitalized patients. For completeness, because of the possible intersection between these addictive agents and the global diabetes epidemic, an account of the growing link between the use of recreational drugs (alcohol, nicotine, marijuana, opioids, cocaine, amphetamine-like drugs and other psychostimulants) and glucose abnormalities has been included.

With some medications, the data presented should help debunk myths, clarify misperceptions, and provide reassurance to practicing clinicians. Wherever the evidence supports increased diabetes risk, clear suggestions are given on how to reduce the risk. Also covered in this book are diabetes management guidelines for special situations, including new-onset diabetes after transplant and TPN-induced hyperglycemia. The final chapter provides a general approach to the prevention or attenuation of diabetes risk, focusing on risk stratification, lifestyle modification, and a critical appraisal of the medications that have been demonstrated, in clinical trials, to prevent or delay diabetes. Also introduced is the emerging concept of diabetes pharmacoprophylaxis in high-risk individuals receiving treatment with potentially diabetogenic agents.

The knowledge gained from reading this book should enable clinicians to become well informed regarding the impact of a wide variety of commonly used medications on glucose homeostasis and the risks of drug-induced diabetes or exacerbation of preexisting diabetes. With such knowledge, clinicians will be better positioned to design and select therapeutic regimens that embody the best risk–benefit profile with regard to glycemia and concurrent management of the primary or comorbid conditions.

1

Overview of Diagnosis, Classification, and Pathophysiology of Diabetes

DIABETES

D
iabetes refers to a group of metabolic disorders that result in hyperglycemia. These disorders have different underlying processes but their common manifestation is hyperglycemia, regardless of underlying process.
More than 29 million Americans have diabetes and approximately 8 million of
these individuals are undiagnosed. Diabetes is a major public health problem
because of the long-term complications (such as blindness, amputations, kidney
failure, heart disease, and stroke) that could occur if the condition is inadequately
controlled. Fortunately, the complications of diabetes can be prevented by main-
taining excellent glycemic control, using comprehensive diabetes management.[1,2]

DIAGNOSIS OF DIABETES AND PREDIABETES

The diagnosis of diabetes (Figure 1.1) can be established using any of the following American Diabetes Association criteria:

- Plasma glucose of ≥126 mg/dL after an overnight fast. A repeat test on a
  different day is required to confirm the diagnosis of diabetes.[3]
- Symptoms of diabetes and a random (nonfasting) plasma glucose of ≥200
  mg/dL.
- A standard oral glucose tolerance test (OGTT) showing a plasma glucose
  level of ≥200 mg/dL at 2 h after ingestion of a 75-g glucose load, provided all testing protocols are followed.
- A hemoglobin A1c level of >6.5%.

In the absence of unequivocal hyperglycemia with typical symptoms, abnormal test results should be confirmed by repeat testing.[3]

Prediabetes

The term *prediabetes* is used to describe persons with impaired glucose tolerance (IGT) or impaired fasting glucose (IFG). IGT is defined by a 2-h OGTT
plasma glucose level >140 mg/dL but <200 mg/dL, and IFG is defined by a fasting plasma glucose level of ≥100 mg/dL but <126 mg/dL.[3] Approximately 86
million Americans have prediabetes, and studies have shown that people with

DOI: 10.2337/9781580406192.01

Criteria for the Diagnosis of Diabetes and Prediabetes			
	Normal	Prediabetes	Diabetes
Fasting Glucose	FPG < 100 mg/dl (<5.6 mM)	100 – 125 mg/dl (5.6-6.9 mM)	FPG ≥ 126 mg/dl (7.0 mM)
OGTT	2-hPG <140mg/dl (<7.8 mM)	140 – 199 mg/dl (7.8-11.0 mM)	≥200 mg/dl (11.1 mM) RBG ≥200 + typical symptoms
HbA1c	HbA1c < 5.7%	5.7 – 6.4%	HbA1c > 6.5%

American Diabetes Association. *Diabetes Care* 2016; 39 (Suppl 1): S13-S22

Figure 1.1—Fasting plasma glucose (FPG), oral glucose tolerance test (OGTT), random blood glucose (RBG), and HbA$_{1c}$ criteria for diagnosis of diabetes and prediabetes.

prediabetes tend to develop type 2 diabetes (T2D) at a rate of ~10% per year. Recently, it was observed that initially normoglycemic offspring of parents with T2D develop incident prediabetes at a rate of ~10% per year.[4] Lifestyle modifications (dietary restriction and exercise) and certain medications can prevent the development of diabetes in people with prediabetes.[5]

Classification of Diabetes

Type 1 diabetes (T1D) accounts for <10% of all cases of diabetes, occurs in younger people, and is caused by absolute insulin deficiency resulting from an immune-mediated destruction of the insulin-producing cells of the pancreas, known as β-cells. T2D accounts for >90% of all cases of diabetes (Figure 1.2). Usually a disease of adults, T2D is being diagnosed increasingly in younger age-groups. Obesity, insulin resistance, and relative insulin deficiency are characteristic findings. Insulin resistance refers to a decreased ability of insulin to drive the uptake of glucose from the blood into the cells and to produce the other appropriate metabolic effects of insulin. People with insulin resistance alone do not develop diabetes, because their pancreatic β-cells compensate by increasing insulin secretion to levels that can maintain normoglycemia. Therefore, a second defect—an inability to maintain compensatory hyperinsulinemia—is required to precipitate T2D. Other specific types of diabetes include those that result from surgical resection or diseases of the exocrine pancreas (such as cystic fibrosis), glandular disorders (e.g., Cushing's syndrome, acromegaly), and monogenic syndromes (e.g., maturity-onset diabetes of the young). Gestational diabetes occurs during the second half of pregnancy and tends to resolve once the baby and placenta have been delivered (although the mother remains at high risk for future T2D).[3]

The Genetic Basis of Diabetes

Interactions between genetic and environmental factors are well recognized in the pathogenesis of T1D and T2D (Figure 1.3). In T1D, the expression of inherited disease susceptibility markers of the major histocompatibility (HLA) gene family predisposes individuals to islet β-cell damage, classically through

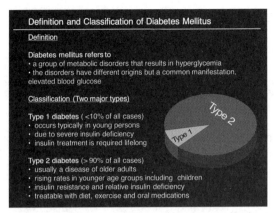

Figure 1.2—The two major types of diabetes mellitus.

autoimmune-mediated mechanisms. The environmental triggers for such auto-immune destruction of the β-cells are believed to include certain viruses.[6] A family history of diabetes in first-degree relatives (parents, siblings, and offspring) is one of the strongest risk factors for the development of diabetes. The genetic transmission of diabetes risk from parents to offspring is rather complex, however, and familial concordance is stronger for T2D than T1D. Among monozygotic (identical) twins, the concordance rate of T2D is ~80%, and the lifetime risk of development of T2D among offspring and siblings of affected patients has been estimated at ~40%.[7] If both parents are affected the risk approaches 80% in offspring.[8] Current understanding indicates that multiple genes are involved in this process, and rarely have single genes been discovered that explained the entire processes underlying the development of diabetes.[9,10]

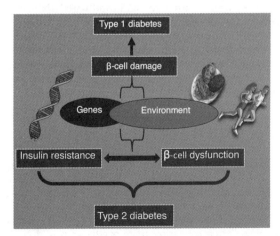

Figure 1.3—Genetic and environmental interactions in the pathophysiology of type 1 and type 2 diabetes. *Source:* Adapted from Dagogo-Jack.[10]

Pathophysiology of Type 2 Diabetes

In genetically susceptible persons, the development of T2D is characterized ultimately by three underlying mechanisms: impaired insulin action (also known as insulin resistance), which is expressed in skeletal muscle and fat cells; impaired insulin secretion by the pancreatic β-cells; and increased hepatic (liver) glucose production (HGP).[11–13] The transition from normal glucose regulation to T2D is punctuated by a variable interlude (usually lasting several years) in the intermediate state of prediabetes (IGT and IFG).

There is general agreement that insulin resistance and impaired insulin secretion are present in most individuals before the onset of diabetes.[12] Longitudinal studies in which initially healthy Pima Indians (a population that has the highest known prevalence of T2D) underwent metabolic assessments repeatedly over several years showed that subjects who progressed from the normal state to prediabetes (IGT) had lost ~12% of their insulin sensitivity but 27% of their insulin secretion; the further progression from prediabetes to T2D was preceded by a 31% decline in insulin sensitivity and a 78% decline in insulin secretion.[14]

DEMOGRAPHIC FACTORS

Age

In 2012, the Centers for Disease Control and Prevention (CDC) estimated that about 208,000 people <20 years old had diagnosed diabetes (T1D or T2D). This represents 0.25% of all people <20 years of age, a sharp contrast from the 25.9% prevalence of diabetes among Americans ≥65 years old.[15] The *SEARCH for Diabetes in Youth*, a multicenter study funded by CDC and the National Institutes of Health (NIH), found that in 2008–2009, an estimated 18,436 people <20 years old in the U.S. were newly diagnosed with T1D annually, and 5,089 people <20 years old were newly diagnosed with T2D annually. Although still uncommon, the rates of new cases of T2D were greater among people age 10–19 years old than in younger children. In national surveys and epidemiological studies, older age always emerges as a robust risk factor for the development of T2D.[16,17]

Gender

The global prevalence of diabetes is fairly balanced by gender.[18,19] During the evolution of T2D, male preponderance occurs at the stage of prediabetes: this has been reported in two cross-sectional surveys (the National Health and Nutrition Examination Survey [NHANES] 1999–2002 and 2005–2006)[20,21] and in the prospective Pathobiology of Prediabetes in a Biracial Cohort (POP-ABC) study.[4] [AU: Please confirm correct reference number.] The lack of a major gender difference among people who eventually develop T2D indicates that gender equilibration occurs during transition from prediabetes to T2D.[22]

Race and Ethnicity

The markedly high prevalence of T2D in Pima Indians (~50% by ≥35 years old) has been noted for a long time.[23] Cross-sectional national surveys also have reported higher prevalence rates of T2D among African Americans, Hispanic Americans, and other ethnic minority groups as compared with non-Hispanic whites.[24–28] However, prospective studies of individuals with prediabetes showed no racial or ethnic differences in progression from prediabetes to T2D during 3 years[5] or 9 years[29] of follow-up. Similarly, in the SHIELD study, race and ethnicity was not a significant predictor of incident diabetes among initially normoglycemic persons followed for ~5 years.[30] In the POP-ABC study, initially normoglycemic African Americans and European Americans with parental history of T2D developed incident prediabetes at a similar rate.[4]

Much of the racial and ethnic demographic information on prevalent diabetes in the U.S. was generated from cross-sectional survey data that relied on self-report during telephone interviews. In the 2005–2006 NHANES,[21] 516 persons who reported having ever been told by a health care professional that they have diabetes were classified as having "diagnosed diabetes," and 3,107 persons who did not report preexisting diabetes underwent evaluation with blood glucose measurements, to estimate the prevalence of undiagnosed diabetes and prediabetes. Among adults 20 years or older, the self-reported prevalence of diagnosed diabetes was 12.8% in non-Hispanic blacks, 8.4% in Mexican Americans, and 6.6% in non-Hispanic whites.[21,28] In contrast, the prevalence of undiagnosed diabetes and that of prediabetes, both of which were based on measured fasting and 2-h post-OGTT plasma glucose values, showed no significant racial or ethnic differences.[21,28]

Thus, national data based on blood glucose measurements are in discord with the twofold black–white difference in self-reported diagnosed diabetes. In fact, these data show lower values for measured fasting and 2-h post-OGTT plasma glucose levels in African Americans compared with white persons.[17,21,28] Furthermore, results of the prospective SHIELD study showed that race or ethnicity was not a significant predictor of incident T2D during 5 years of follow-up of a diverse cohort of initially normoglycemic subjects.[31] The recent use of HbA$_{1c}$ for diagnosis probably inflates the magnitude of racial and ethnic differences in the prevalence of diabetes and prediabetes, as ethnic differences in HbA$_{1c}$ values may be explained, at least in part, by nonglycemic factors.[16,32,33]

Genetic and environmental risk factors contribute to diabetes susceptibility in different populations (Figure 1.3 and Table 1.1).[34] The evidence, however, for significant racial differences in major diabetes risk alleles of genome-wide significance has not been compelling.[9,10] Thus, no clear biological mechanisms explain why objective estimates of undiagnosed diabetes would follow a different racial pattern from that of self-reported prevalence of diagnosed diabetes. Undoubtedly, among people with diagnosed diabetes in the U.S., there are marked ethnic disparities in the quality of diabetes control and complications from diabetes. It is most likely that suboptimal glycemic control, rather than race or ethnicity per se, underlies much of the greater burden of diabetes complications among U.S. ethnic minority populations.[32,34,35]

Table 1.1—Risk Factors for Type 2 Diabetes

■ Genetic, familial, race/ethnicity

■ Increasing age

■ Being overweight or obese

■ Habitual physical inactivity

■ Having dyslipidemia (elevated triglycerides or decreased HDL cholesterol)

■ Having hypertension

■ History of gestational diabetes or birth of child weighing 9 lb or more

■ History of polycystic ovary syndrome

■ History of vascular disease

■ History of impaired fasting glucose or impaired glucose tolerance

INSULIN RESISTANCE

The binding of insulin to its receptor triggers a series of phosphorylation reactions in the cytosol. The initial phosphorylation occurs on tyrosine residues within the cytoplasmic tail of the insulin receptor, followed by phosphorylation of multiple other intracellular proteins, including insulin receptor substrates (IRS)-1, 2, 3, and 4. In insulin-sensitive tissues (skeletal muscle and adipose), phosphorylation of the IRS proteins activates the enzyme phosphatidylinositol 3-kinase (PI3-kinase), leading to downstream activation of Akt/protein kinase B (PKB) and the translocation of an intracellular pool of glucose transporter molecules (GLUT4) to the plasma membrane, where they form vesicles that mediate glucose transport into the cell (Figure 1.4). Thus, insulin lowers blood glucose by stimulating the

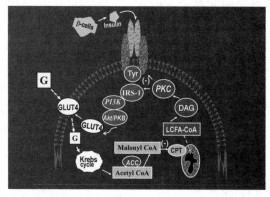

Figure 1.4—Schema showing insulin signaling and interactions with glucose (G) and fatty acid metabolism.

transport of glucose across cell membranes through a series of complex chemical reactions. Failure of this mechanism at any level between the binding of insulin to its cell membrane receptor and the eventual translocation of GLUT4 and internalization of glucose results in insulin resistance. Phosphorylation of serine or threonine residues (instead of tyrosine) interferes with insulin signaling, and is a common molecular mechanism that leads to insulin resistance.

Insulin resistance can be inherited or acquired. Obesity, aging, physical inactivity, overeating, and accumulation of nonestrified (free) fatty acids (NEFAs) are known causes of insulin resistance. Normally, cytoplasmic NEFAs in the form of long-chain fatty acyl coenzyme A (LCFA-CoA) are transported into mitochondria for β-oxidation, a process that is gated by carnitine palmitoyl transferase (CPT)-1 and CPT-2 (the shuttle enzymes located in the outer and inner mitochdrial membrane; Figure 1.4). This shuttle process ensures that NEFAs do not accumulate excessively in the cytoplasm. Inhibition of that process leads to the accumulation of LCFA-CoA, which can lead to lipotoxicity.[13] Also, intracellular accumulation of fatty acids can activate protein kinase C (PKC) via diacylglycerol (DAG), leading to aberrant phosphorylation at serine or threonine residues instead of tyrosine (Figure 1.4). As noted, serine or threonine phosphorylation produces insulin resistance by short-circuiting the normal insulin signal transduction that leads to GLUT4 translocation and glucose transport into cells. Interestingly, acetyl CoA, a product of glycolysis in the Krebs cycle, can be converted to malonyl CoA by the enzyme acetyl CoA carboxylase (ACC). Malonyl CoA is a potent inhibitor of CPT-1, a process that thwarts mitochondrial fat oxidation and promotes the accumulation of fatty acids in the cytosol.[36] Glucose abundance also increases the formation of intracellular DAG. Thus, multiple metabolic pathways link intracellular glucose abundance (usually derived from carbohydrate consumption) to impaired fat oxidation, cytosolic fat accumulation, risk of lipotoxicity, and insulin resistance (Figure 1.4). Caloric restriction through the reduction of carbohydrate and fat intake has been shown to improve insulin sensitivity and prevent T2D.[37,38]

Increased Lipolysis

As a consequence of insulin resistance in adipocytes, the inhibitory effects of insulin on plasma NEFA levels and adipocyte NEFA turnover are markedly impaired.[13,39,40] The net effect is increased lipolysis and NEFA turnover in the setting of insulin resistance. Thus, patients with T2D are exposed to chronic elevation in plasma NEFA levels, which leads to increased gluconeogenesis, exacerbation of insulin resistance in hepatocytes and myocytes, and impairment of insulin secretion.[41,42] Furthermore, a morphological shift to a larger adipocyte size occurs in the setting of insulin resistance along with aberrant adipocyte function, resulting in the increased secretion of proinflammatory molecules and decreased production of adiponectin, a protective adipocytokine. Notably, the enlarged adipocytes in insulin-resistant subjects have a reduced capacity for storing fat, which causes excessive lipid deposition at ectopic sites, such as muscle, liver, β-cells, and vascular smooth cells.[13,43] As noted, the intracellular accumulation of fatty acids leads to lipotoxicity, with dire consequences for cellular function, insulin sensitivity, and insulin secretion.[13]

Insulin Secretion

Under normal conditions, the pancreatic β-cells secrete insulin in response to glucose stimulation through a series of transmembrane electrical reactions. Glucose metabolism in β-cells generates bursts of action potentials that ultimately lead to calcium influx. The adenosine triphosphate (ATP)–sensitive potassium channel (K_{ATP}) normally maintains the β-cell resting membrane potential, thereby preventing calcium entry. The K_{ATP} channel is closed when the ratio of ATP to adenosine diphosphate rises within the β-cells as occurs during glucose metabolism. The resultant depolarization (change in electrical charge) of the β-cell membrane drives calcium into the cell, which then triggers insulin secretion (Figure 1.5). Agents that open the K_{ATP} channel (e.g., diazoxide) reverse the depolarization and inhibit insulin secretion by the β-cells. The β-cell mass is reduced in T2D patients because of apoptosis induced by toxic islet amyloid, oxidative stress, inflammatory cytokines, and other mechanisms.[44-46]

Hepatic Glucose Production

In the prospective study of Pima Indians, HGP remained normal during the transition from normal glucose tolerance to IGT, but increased by 15% with further progression to T2D.[14] In patients with established T2D, the rate of hepatic gluconeogenesis is not suppressed postprandially (as occurs normally). Thus, the upregulated HGP becomes a key determinant of fasting as well as postprandial glucose excursions in T2D. The increased HGP is triggered by an increased flux of lipolytic products and other glucose precursors and is exacerbated by hepatic insulin resistance.

Glucagon and Incretins

Glucagon hypersecretion by the pancreatic α-cells is a characteristic of both T1D and T2D.[47] The hyperglucagonemia in patients with diabetes is particu-

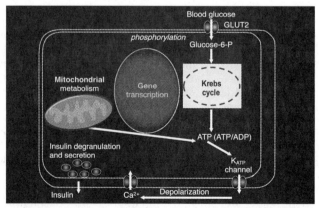

Figure 1.5—Process of glucose-stimulated insulin secretion by the pancreatic β-cell.

larly inappropriate in the postprandial period when glucon levels are expected to be suppressed. The failure of postprandial glucagon suppression in patients with T1D and T2D results from loss of pulsatile intraislet insulin secretion and leads to exaggerated postprandial glucose excursions.[48] Autopsy studies in patients with T2D further show preservation of α-cell mass, despite marked depletion of β-cell mass.[44] Incretin hormones (glucagon-like peptide [GLP]-1 and glucose-dependent insulinotropic peptide [GIP]), normally secreted by the enterocytes in response to food, amplify postprandial insulin secretion and suppress glucagon secretion. Emerging data indicate that T2D is associated with impaired incretin secretion and relative resistance to the action of incretin hormones. The major pathophysiological defects in T2D are summarized in Figure 1.6.[13]

Renal Glucose Reabsorption

Under normal conditions, ~180 g of glucose are filtered by the glomerulus, but no glycosuria ensues because of efficient reabsorption by renal tubules. Renal tubular glucose reabsorption is mediated by specialized adluminal sodium glucose cotransporters (SGLT)-1 and SGLT2 (the latter being the major transporter) and basolateral glucose transporters GLUT1 and GLUT2 molecules. In patients with diabetes, hyperglycemia exceeds renal tubular maximum, leading to glycosuria commensurate with the degree of hyperglycemia. Mutations in the SGLT2 gene have been described in patients with familial renal glycosuria, a benign condition that is not associated with diabetes or hyperglycemia.[49] It appears that renal glucose reabsorption may be inappropriately efficient in the setting of hyperglycemia and that SGLT2, GLUT1, and GLUT2 may be upregulated in the kidney of patients with T2D.[13,50,51] Indeed, several SGLT2 inhibitors have now been approved for the treatment of T2D and are effective in decreasing hyperglycemia by promoting renal glucose excretion.

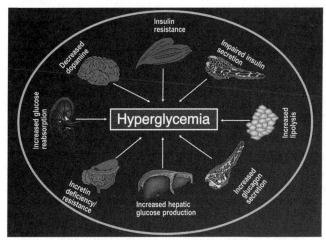

Figure 1.6—Major pathophysiological defects in type 2 diabetes.

Central Dopaminergic Pathways

Emerging data indicate that central nervous system dopaminergic pathways modulate food intake, and glucose, energy, and weight homeostasis. Decreased dopaminergic tone and polymorphisms of the dopamine D2 receptor are associated with increased risks of obesity and T2D.[52,53] Conversely, augmentation of dopaminergic activity has been shown to improve glucose tolerance and insulin sensitivity, reduce adiposity, and improve lipid profile.[54,55] A quick-release form of bromocriptine (BQR) has been approved for the treatment of T2D on the basis of its ability to "reset" central dopaminergic tone and improve related neurotransmission pathways.[56] An ancillary mechanism of action of BQR may be its ability to reduce adrenergic tone, thus mitigating adrenergic-related increase in insulin resistance, glucose, and blood pressure.[56,57]

CONCLUSION

Current understanding indicates that multiple pathophysiological defects underlie T2D. The exact sequence of evolution of individual defects has not been determined precisely; many of the defects coevolve during the pathogenesis of T2D and are demonstrable even at the stage of prediabetes (Figure 1.6).[4,11,13,14]

REFERENCES

1. DCCT/EDIC Research Group. Modern-day clinical course of type 1 diabetes mellitus after 30 years' duration: the Diabetes Control and Complications Trial/Epidemiology of Diabetes Interventions and Complications and Pittsburgh epidemiology of diabetes complications experience (1983–2005). *Arch Intern Med* 2009;169:1307–1316

2. UK Prospective Diabetes Study (UKPDS) Group. Intensive blood-glucose control with sulphonylureas or insulin compared with conventional treatment and risk of complications in patients with type 2 diabetes (UKPDS 33). *Lancet* 1998;352:837–853

3. American Diabetes Association. Standards of medical care in diabetes–2016. *Diabetes Care* 2015;39(Suppl. 1):S4–S104

4. Dagogo-Jack S, Edeoga C, Ebenibo S, Nyenwe E, Wan J; for the Pathobiology of Prediabetes in a Biracial Cohort (POP-ABC) Research Group. Lack of racial disparity in incident prediabetes and glycemic progression among black and white offspring of parents with type 2 diabetes: the Pathobiology of Prediabetes in a Biracial Cohort (POP-ABC) Study. *J Clin Endocrinol* 2014;99:E1078–E1087

5. Diabetes Prevention Program Research Group. Reduction in the incidence of type 2 diabetes with lifestyle intervention or metformin. *N Engl J Med* 2002;346:393–403

6. Atkinson MA, Eisenbarth GS, Michels AW. Type 1 diabetes. *Lancet* 2014;383:69–82

7. Granner DK, O'Brien RM. Molecular physiology and genetics of NIDDM. *Diabetes Care* 1992;15:369–388

8. Martin BC, Warram JH, Krolewski AS, Bergman RN, Soeldner JS, Kahn CR. Role of glucose and insulin resistance in the development of type 2 diabetes mellitus: results of a 25-year follow-up study. *Lancet* 1992;340:925–929

9. Hivert MF, Jablonski KA, Perreault L, Saxena R, McAteer JB, Franks PW, Hamman RF, Kahn SE, Haffner S; DIAGRAM Consortium, Meigs JB, Altshuler D, Knowler WC, Florez JC; Diabetes Prevention Program Research Group. Updated genetic score based on 34 confirmed type 2 diabetes loci is associated with diabetes incidence and regression to normoglycemia in the Diabetes Prevention Program. *Diabetes* 2011;60:1340–1348

10. Dagogo-Jack S. Predicting diabetes: our relentless quest for genomic nuggets. *Diabetes Care* 2012;35:193–195

11. Dagogo-Jack S, Santiago JV. Pathophysiology of type 2 diabetes and modes of action of therapeutic interventions. *Arch Intern Med* 1997;157:1802–1817

12. Moneva M, Dagogo-Jack S. Multiple drug targets in the management of type 2 diabetes mellitus. *Current Drug Targets* 2002;3:203–221

13a. Defronzo RA. Banting Lecture. From the triumvirate to the ominous octet: a new paradigm for the treatment of type 2 diabetes mellitus. *Diabetes* 2009;58:773–795

13b. DeFronzo RA. Insulin resistance, lipotoxicity, type 2 diabetes and atherosclerosis: the missing links. The Claude Bernard Lecture 2009. *Diabetologia* 2010;53:1270–1287

14. Weyer C, Bogardus C, Mott DM, Pratley R. The natural history of insulin secretory dysfunction and insulin resistance in the pathogenesis of type 2 diabetes mellitus. *J Clin Invest* 1999;104:787–794

15. Centers for Disease Control and Prevention. National diabetes statistics report, 2014. Available from http://www.cdc.gov/diabetes/pubs/statsreport14/national-diabetes-report-web.pdf. Accessed 5 January 2016

16. Cowie CC, Rust KF, Byrd-Holt DD, Gregg EW, Ford ES, Geiss LS, Bainbridge KE, Fradkin JE. Prevalence of diabetes and high risk for diabetes using A1C criteria in the U.S. population in 1988–2006. *Diabetes Care* 2010;33:562–568

17. Menke A, Rust KF, Savage PJ, Cowie CC. Hemoglobin A1c, fasting plasma glucose, and 2-hour plasma glucose distributions in US population subgroups: NHANES 2005–2010. *Ann Epidemiol* 2014;24:83–89

18. Gale EA, Gillespie KM. Diabetes and gender. *Diabetologia* 200;44:3–15

19. Wild S, Roglic G, Green A, Sicree R, King H. Global prevalence of diabetes: estimates for the year 2000 and projections for 2030. *Diabetes Care* 2004;27:1047–1053

20. Centers for Disease Control and Prevention. National Health Interview Survey (NHIS). Available from http://www.cdc.gov/nchs/nhis.htm. Accessed 5 July 2015

21. Centers for Disease Control and Prevention. 2008 National Center for Health Statistics: National Health and Nutrition Examination Survey 2005–2006, 2008. Available from http://www.cdc.gov/nchs/about/major/nhanes/nhanes2005-2006/nhanes05_06.htm. Accessed 5 July 2015

22. Perreault L, Ma Y, Dagogo-Jack S, Horton E, Marrero D, Crandall J, Barrett-Connor E; Diabetes Prevention Program. Sex differences in diabetes risk and the effect of intensive lifestyle modification in the Diabetes Prevention Program. *Diabetes Care* 2008;31:1416–1421

23. Knowler WC, Bennett PH, Hamman RF, Miller M. Diabetes incidence and prevalence in Pima Indians: a 19-fold greater incidence than in Rochester, Minnesota. *Am J Epidemiol* 1978;108:497–505

24. Centers for Disease Control and Prevention. 2011 National diabetes fact sheet. Diagnosed and undiagnosed diabetes in the United States, all ages, 2010. Available from http://www.cdc.gov/diabetes/pubs/estimates11.htm. Accessed 5 July 2015

25. Brancati FL, Kao WH, Folsom AR, Watson RL, Szklo M. Incident type 2 diabetes mellitus in African American and white adults: the Atherosclerosis Risk in Communities Study. *JAMA* 2000;283:2253–2259

26. Harris MI. Racial and ethnic differences in health care access and health outcomes for adults with type 2 diabetes. *Diabetes Care* 2001;24:454–459

27. Cowie CC, Rust KF, Byrd-Holt DD, Eberhardt MS, Flegal KM, Engelgau MM, Saydah SH, Williams DE, Geiss LS, Gregg EW. Prevalence of diabetes and impaired fasting glucose in adults in the U.S. population: National Health and Nutrition Examination Survey 1999–2002. *Diabetes Care* 2006;29:1263–1268

28. Cowie CC, Rust KF, Ford ES, Eberhardt MS, Byrd-Holt DD, Li C, Williams DE, Gregg EW, Bainbridge KE, Saydah SH, Geiss LS. Full accounting of diabetes and pre-diabetes in the U.S. population in 1988–1994 and 2005–2006. *Diabetes Care* 2009;32:287–294

29. Diabetes Prevention Program Research Group. 10-year follow-up of diabetes incidence and weight loss in the Diabetes Prevention Program Outcomes Study. *Lancet* 2009;374:1677–1686

30. Rodbard HW, Bays HE, Gavin JR 3rd, et al. Rate and risk predictors for development of self-reported type-2 diabetes mellitus over a 5-year period: the SHIELD study. *Int J Clin Pract* 2012;66:684–691

31. Rodbard HW, Bays HE, Gavin JR 3rd, Green AJ, Bazata DD, Lewis SJ, Fox KM, Reed ML, Grandy S. Rate and risk predictors for development of self-reported type-2 diabetes mellitus over a 5-year period: the SHIELD study. *Int J Clin Pract* 2012;66:684–691

32. Selvin E, Parrinello CM, Sacks DB, Coresh J. Trends in prevalence and control of diabetes in the U.S., 1988–1994 and 1999–2010. *Ann Intern Med* 2014;160:517–525

33. Dagogo-Jack S. Pitfalls in the use of HbA1c as a diagnostic test: the ethnic conundrum. *Nat Rev Endocrinol* 2010;6:589–593

34. Egede LE, Dagogo-Jack S. Epidemiology of type 2 diabetes: focus on ethnic minorities. *Med Clin N Am* 2005;89:949–975

35. Karter AJ, Ferrara A, Liu JY, Moffet HH, Ackerson LM, Selby JV. Ethnic disparities in diabetic complications in an insured population. *JAMA* 2002;287:2519–2527

36. Rasmussen BB, Holmbäck UC, Volpi E, et al. Malonyl coenzyme A and the regulation of functional carnitine palmitoyltransferase-1 activity and fat oxidation in human skeletal muscle. *J Clin Invest* 2002;110:1687–1693

37. Kitabchi AE, Temprosa M, Knowler WC, et al. Role of insulin secretion and sensitivity in the evolution of type 2 diabetes in the Diabetes Prevention Program: effects of lifestyle intervention and metformin. *Diabetes* 2005;54:2404–2414

38. Larson-Meyer DE, Heilbronn LK, Redman LM, et al. Effect of calorie restriction with or without exercise on insulin sensitivity, β-cell function, fat cell size, and ectopic lipid in overweight subjects. *Diabetes Care* 2006;29:1337–1344

39. Groop LC, Bonadonna RC, Del Prato S, Ratheiser K, Zyck K, DeFronzo RA. Glucose and free fatty acid metabolism in non-insulin-dependent diabetes mellitus: evidence for multiple sites of insulin resistance. *J Clin Invest* 1989;84:205–213

40. Groop LC, Saloranta C, Shank M, Bonadonna RC, Ferrannini E, DeFronzo RA. The role of free fatty acid metabolism in the pathogenesis of insulin resistance in obesity and noninsulin-dependent diabetes mellitus. *J Clin Endocrinol Metab* 1991;72:96-107

41. Roden M, Price TB, Perseghin G, Petersen KF, Rothman DL, Cline GW, Shulman GI. Mechanism of free fatty acid-induced insulin resistance in humans. *J Clin Invest* 1996;97:2859–2865

42. Carpentier A, Mittelman SD, Bergman RN, Giacca A, Lewis GF. Prolonged elevation of plasma free fatty acids impairs pancreatic β-cell function in obese nondiabetic humans but not in individuals with type 2 diabetes. *Diabetes* 2000;49:399–408

43. Bray GA, Glennon JA, Salans LB, Horton ES, Danforth E Jr, Sims EA. Spontaneous and experimental human obesity: effects of diet and adipose cell size on lipolysis and lipogenesis. *Metabolism* 1977;26:739–747

44. Clark A, Wells CA, Buley ID, Cruickshank JK, Vanhegan RI, Matthews DR, Cooper GJ, Holman RR, Turner RC. Islet amyloid, increased A-cells, reduced B-cells and exocrine fibrosis: quantitative changes in the pancreas in type 2 diabetes. *Diabetes Res* 1988;9:151–159

45. Haataja L, Gurlo T, Huang CJ, Butler PC. Islet amyloid in type 2 diabetes, and the toxic oligomer hypothesis. *Endocr Rev* 2008;29:303–316

46. Butler AE, Janson J, Bonner-Weir S, Ritzel R, Rizza RA, Butler PC. B-cell deficit and increased β-cell apoptosis in humans with type 2 diabetes. *Diabetes* 2003;52:102–110

47. Unger RH, Aguilar-Parada E, Muller WA, Eisentraut AM. Studies of pancreatic alpha cell function in normal and diabetic subjects. *J Clin Invest* 1970;49:837–848

48. Meier JJ, Kjems LL, Veldhuis JD, et al. Postprandial suppression of glucagon secretion depends on intact pulsatile insulin secretion: further evidence for the intraislet insulin hypothesis. *Diabetes* 2006;55:1051–1056

49. Santer R, Kinner M, Lassen CL, Schneppenheim R, Eggert P, Bald M, Brodehl J, Daschner M, Ehrich JH, Kemper M, Li Volti S, Neuhaus T, Skovby F, Swift PG, Schaub J, Klaerke D. Molecular analysis of the SGLT2 gene in patients with renal glucosuria. *J Am Soc Nephrol* 2003;14:2873–2882

50. Rahmoune H, Thompson PW, Ward JM, Smith CD, Hong G, Brown J. Glucose transporters in human renal proximal tubular cells isolated from the urine of patients with non-insulin-dependent diabetes. *Diabetes* 2005;54:3427–3434

51. Bakris GL, Fonseca VA, Sharma K, Wright EM. Renal sodium-glucose transport: role in diabetes mellitus and potential clinical implications. *Kidney Int* 2009;75:1272–1277

52. Cincotta AH, Meier AH. Bromocriptine inhibits in vivo free fatty acid oxidation and hepatic glucose output in seasonally obese hamsters (Mesocricetus auratus). *Metabolism* 1995;44:1349–1355

53. Barnard ND, Noble EP, Ritchie T, et al. D2 dopamine receptor Taq1A polymorphism, body weight, and dietary intake in type 2 diabetes. *Nutrition* 2009;25:58–65

54. Cincotta AH, Tozzo E, Scislowski PW. Bromocriptine/SKF38393 treatment ameliorates obesity and associated metabolic dysfunctions in obese (ob/ob) mice. *Life Sci* 1997;61:951–956

55. Pijl H, Ohashi S, Matsuda M, Miyazaki Y, Mahankali A, Kumar V, Pipek R, Iozzo P, Lancaster JL, Cincotta AH, DeFronzo RA. Bromocriptine: a novel approach to the treatment of type 2 diabetes. *Diabetes Care* 2000;23:1154–1161

56. Gaziano JM, Cincotta AH, Vinik A, Blonde L, Bohannon N, Scranton R. Effect of bromocriptine-QR (a quick-release formulation of bromocriptine mesylate) on major adverse cardiovascular events in type 2 diabetes subjects. *J Am Heart Assoc* 2012;1(5):e002279. doi: 10.1161/JAHA.112.002279. Epub 2012 Oct 25

57. Garber AJ, Blonde L, Bloomgarden JT, Dagogo-Jack S. Bromocriptine-QR for type 2 diabetes: AACE Expert Panel review of its potential place in therapy. *Endocr Pract* 2013;19:100–106

2

Medications and Diabetes Risk: General Mechanisms

iabetes has been reported in association with exposure to a wide variety of medications. As summarized in Table 2.1, in many cases, the mechanism relating the particular drug to hyperglycemia is explainable, whereas the mechanism of the association is less clear with regard to several other medications.[1] Classically, elevated blood glucose can result from drugs that induce hypoinsulinemia through the destruction of pancreatic β-cells (e.g., pentamidine, Vacor), or drugs that inhibit insulin secretion (e.g., diazoxide). Hypokalemia impairs insulin secretion and also desensitizes the insulin receptor, and it is one mechanism underlying the dysglycemia associated with thiazides, loop diuretics, and hyperaldosteronism.[2]

The induction of insulin resistance is a classic mechanism for steroid-induced diabetes, but the underlying processes are complex (with contributions from hyperglucagonemia, glycogenolysis, lipolysis, and gluconeogenesis). Even in the

Table 2.1—Mechanisms and Examples of Drug-Induced Hyperglycemia

Mechanisms	Examples
A. Interference with insulin secretion	Diazoxide, β-blockers
	Diuretics
Pancreatotoxic	Pentamidine, Vacor
B. Interference with insulin action	Diuretics (via hypokalemia)
	Glucocorticoids, antiretrovirals
	β-Agonists, growth hormone
C. Impaired insulin secretion and action	Thiazide diuretics
	Cyclosporin, Tacrolimus
D. Increased nutrient flux and gluconeogenesis	Nicotinic acid
	Total parenteral nutrition
	α-Interferon
E. Alteration of gut flora	Antibiotics?
F. Unknown mechanism	Nonsteroidal anti-inflammatory drugs
	Antipsychotics
	Antidepressants

DOI: 10.2337/9781580406192.02

setting of astronomical insulin resistance, a failure of compensatory insulin secretion must be held as a permissive factor for any resultant hyperglycemia. Besides the classical mechanisms of insulin resistance and β-cell dysfunction, other factors, such as alteration of blood flow and intestinal microbial flora, have been proposed in the etiology of drug-associated diabetes.[3] As argued, drugs that restrict blood flow impair the normal delivery of substrates to insulin-sensitive tissues (especially, skeletal muscle) and, via that mechanism, could reduce glucose disposal and promote hyperglycemia.[4] Theoretically, vasoconstrictors and β-blockers (unopposed α-adrenergic activity) could induce dysglycemia through that mechanism. In many instances, multiple mechanisms, including unknown factors, appear to mediate the effects of drugs on glucose metabolism. It is important to recognize drug-induced diabetes as soon as possible, because withdrawal of the offending drug (if clinically feasible and appropriate) should result in prompt resolution of the diabetes, in the absence of permanent cellular damage to the insulin-secreting β-cells.

RISK FACTOR VERSUS CAUSATION: THE BRADFORD HILL'S CRITERIA

Originally established by Sir Austin Bradford Hill[5] and later elaborated by others, Hill's criteria form the basis of establishing scientifically valid causal connections between potential disease agents and the many diseases that afflict humankind. The criteria are as follows: *1)* temporal relationship, an essential requirement that exposure to the agent must necessarily always precede the occurrence of the disease; *2)* strength of association; *3)* dose response, a requirement that exposure to increasing amounts of the agent should result in increasing severity of disease; *4)* consistency; *5)* biological plausibility, with regard to currently accepted understanding of disease mechanisms; *6)* consideration of alternate explanations; *7)* experimental insight, a requirement that the observed association be reproducible and modifiable through deliberate experimentation; *8)* specificity of the association; and *9)* coherence, which requires that the association be compatible with existing theory and knowledge.

Applying Hill's criteria,[5] only a few exceptions (e.g., pancreatic toxins and steroid-induced diabetes), among the myriad of medications that have been reported to alter blood glucose levels, meet the scientific threshold for establishing direct causality. For the majority of medications, the occurrence of diabetes is observed only in a minority of patients exposed, and the reported link to diabetes suffers from the paucity of data from randomized controlled studies, weak association, inconsistent pattern, indeterminate temporal relationship (resulting from lack of baseline glucose data in many cases), unclear mechanisms, and uncertain dose-response relationship.

Despite these caveats, it behooves clinicians to keep an open mind and maintain vigilance, because the lack of gold-standard evidence of causation may not be absolute evidence of the lack of a possible causal relationship. A case in point is the relationship between smoking and diseases of the lung and heart. No randomized controlled trials, in which subjects are allocated to smoke cigarettes or placebo "cigarettes" and are followed for many years until the development of lung or heart disease, can ever be conceived let alone conducted for obvious ethical and moral reasons. As a result, the epidemiological and association studies have held sway, such that their results demonstrating strong, consistent, and dose-response relationships between smoking and several cardiopulmonary disorders have informed the promulgation of far-reaching antismoking measures.[6]

Besides a direct, causal mechanism, possible explanations for treatment-emergent diabetes could include preexisting undiagnosed diabetes; increased susceptibility to diabetes from underlying genetic or environmental risk factors; an indirect effect mediated by known risk factors, such as weight gain; a coincidental finding; or an idiosyncratic reaction in susceptible persons that is inherently unpredictable.

DRUGS ASSOCIATED WITH TYPE 1 DIABETES

Type 1 diabetes (T1D) is a disease of absolute or severe insulin deficiency. The vast majority of patients with T1D have autoimmune destruction of the pancreatic islet β-cells as the underlying mechanism for the insulin deficiency. In a small minority of patients with T1D, evidence for autoimmunity is lacking and the etiology of islet destruction is unclear. Drug-induced T1D is rare in clinical practice. Experimental insulin-deficient diabetes can be induced by treating rodents with the pancreatic toxins streptozotocin or alloxan. Ingestion of the rat poison Vacor (N-3 pyridylmethyl-N' 4 nitrophenyl urea), which is structurally related to alloxan and streptozotocin, has been associated with human cases of diabetes.[7,8] The diabetes induced by Vacor poisoning can have a delayed onset (≥1 week), but it usually is severe and often presents with ketoacidosis. Prophylactic treatment with the antidote nicotinamide should be started as soon as possible following ingestion of Vacor, even in euglycemic persons.[7,9]

The antiprotozoal drug pentamidine, widely used for the treatment of refractory Pneumocystis jirovecii pneumonia (PJP; formerly known as Pneumocystis carinii pneumonia [PCP]) in HIV-infected patients and transplant recipients, can induce acute insulinopenic diabetes in some patients through destruction of the pancreatic β-cells.[10,11] An initial phase of hypoglycemia (reflecting β-cell degranulation and transient hyperinsulinemia) may precede the development of pentamidine-induced diabetes.[12]

The risk factors and exact mechanisms for β-cell destruction by pentamidine are unknown, and the resultant diabetes tends to persist after withdrawal of pentamidine.[10] In vitro studies suggest that pentamidine might be a substrate for the organic cation transporter 1 (OCT1).[13] The OCTs modulate the availability of cationic drugs, such as metformin.[14] Interestingly, cimetidine (an inhibitor of OCTs) has been shown to augment pentamidine-induced hyperglycemia in a rat model.[15] The latter finding suggests that hyperglycemia following pentamidine exposure is related to drug availability and could be exacerbated by coadministration of cimetidine and other drugs that inhibit OCT1.

Alcoholism and chronic pancreatitis have been associated with the development of insulin-deficient diabetes.[16] More than 500 individual drugs have been associated with the risk of acute pancreatitis as an adverse effect, yet in only a small percentage of drugs has causality be established.[17] Additionally, it is chronic exocrine pancreatic inflammation and damage rather than acute pancreatitis that is more likely to be linked etiologically to diabetes risk. The subject of alcohol and diabetes risk is discussed further in Chapter 10. It is possible that other as yet unidentified environmental toxins may be involved in the pathogenesis of the rare nonautoimmune cases of T1D.

DRUGS ASSOCIATED WITH TYPE 2 DIABETES

In contrast to the rarity of drug-associated typical T1D, several commonly used medications have been associated with the development of phenotypical type 2 diabetes (T2D). The latter classification is based loosely on the absence of absolute insulinopenia together with evidence for insulin resistance or related mechanisms for the disruption of glucoregulation. Depending on the severity and acuteness of the perturbation, some patients with drug-related diabetes may present with diabetic ketoacidosis (DKA). The fact that DKA is more characteristic of T1D than T2D may lead physicians to classify such presentations as T1D. Note, however, that ~25% of patients with T2D in the general population present with DKA.[18,19] After initial stabilization with insulin therapy and fluid repletion, the majority of such patients respond to oral antidiabetic agents, as is typical of T2D. Therefore, it is more important to stabilize the patient with drug-related hyperglycemic crisis than to be distracted by a quest for an exact classification in the acute setting. In fact, in many instances, the exact mechanism of the medication-related hyperglycemia remains obscure, and the condition is best assigned to the other category.

According to the Centers for Disease Control and Prevention (CDC), the age-adjusted percentage of adults ≥18 years old with diagnosed diabetes who reported having hypertension was 57.1% in 2009.[20] Other chronic comorbidities frequently found in people with diabetes include dyslipidemia, degenerative joint disease, chronic obstructive pulmonary disease, sleep apnea, congestive heart failure, affective disorders, and peptic ulcer disease. People with diabetes also are at risk for infections. These various conditions often require chronic or recurrent treatment with a wide array of medications, some of which could affect insulin sensitivity, β-cell function, or other aspects of glucoregulation. Whenever feasible, preference should be given to those agents that are either neutral or beneficial in their effects on carbohydrate and lipid metabolism.

In the chapters that follow, different classes of medications will be discussed with regard to their impact on diabetes risk. These medication classes were selected for discussion based either on *1)* their historical association with dysglycemia in clinical practice, *2)* extensive utilization for the management of comorbid conditions (e.g., hypertension, dyslipidemia) in patients with diabetes, or *3)* existing or emerging reports of possible association with dysglycemia.

REFERENCES

1. Comi RJ. Drug-induced diabetes mellitus. In *Diabetes Mellitus.* 2nd ed. LeRoith, Taylor, Olefsky, Eds. Lippincott Williams & Wilkins, Philadelphia, 2000, p. 582–588

2. Zillich AJ, Garg J, Basu S, Bakris GL, Carter BL. Thiazide diuretics, potassium, and the development of diabetes: a quantitative review. *Hypertension* 2006;48:219–224

3. Boursi B, Mamtani R, Haynes K, Yang YX. The effect of past antibiotic exposure on diabetes risk. *Eur J Endocrinol* 2015;172:639–648

4. McCullen MK, Ahmed I. Drug-induced hyperglycemia and diabetes mellitus. In *Type 2 Diabetes, Principles and Practice.* 2nd ed. Goldstein BJ and Müller-Wieland D, Eds. Taylor & Francis, New York, 2007, p. 513–528

5. Hill AB. The environment and disease: association or causation? *Proc Royal Soc Med* 1965;58:295–300

6. Jha P, Ramasundarahettige C, Landsman V, Rostron B, Thun M, Anderson RN, McAfee T, Peto R. 21st-century hazards of smoking and benefits of cessation in the United States. *N Engl J Med* 2013;368:341–350

7. Miller LV, Stokes JD, Silpipat C. Diabetes mellitus and autonomic dysfunction after vacor rodenticide ingestion. *Diabetes Care* 1978;1:73–76

8. Pont A, Rubino JM, Bishop D, Peal R. Diabetes mellitus and neuropathy following vacor ingestion in man. *Arch Intern Med* 1979;139:185–187

9. LeWitt PA. The neurotoxicity of the rat poison vacor. A clinical study of 12 cases. *N Engl J Med* 1980;302:73–77

10. Liegl U, Bogner JR, Goebel FD. Insulin-dependent diabetes mellitus following pentamidine therapy in a patient with AIDS. *Clin Investig* 1994;72:1027–1029

11. Coyle P, Carr AD, Depczynski BB, Chisholm DJ. Diabetes mellitus associated with pentamidine use in HIV-infected patients. *Med J Aust* 1996;165:587–588

12. Bouchard Ph, Saï P, Reach G, Caubarrere I, Ganeval D, Assan R. Diabetes mellitus following pentamidine-induced hypoglycemia in humans. *Diabetes* 1982;31:40–45

13. Jung N, Lehmann C, Rubbert A, Knispel M, Hartmann P, van Lunzen J, Stellbrink HJ, Faetkenheuer G, Taubert D. Relevance of the organic cation transporters 1 and 2 for antiretroviral drug therapy in human immunodeficiency virus infection. *Drug Metab Dispos* 2008;36:1616–1623

14. Wang DS, Jonker JW, Kato Y, Kusuhara H, Schinkel AH, Sugiyama Y. Involvement of organic cation transporter 1 in hepatic and intestinal distribution of metformin. *J Pharmacol Exp Ther* 2002;302:510–515

15. Arino TI, Karakawa S, Ishiwata Y, Nagata M, Yasuhara M. Effect of cimetidine on pentamidine induced hyperglycemia in rats. *Eur J Pharmacol* 2012;693:72–79

16. Ito T, Otsuki M, Itoi T, Shimosegawa T, Funakoshi A, Shiratori K, Naruse S, Kuroda Y; Research Committee of Intractable Diseases of the Pancreas. Pancreatic diabetes in a follow-up survey of chronic pancreatitis in Japan. *J Gastroenterol* 2007;42:291–297

17. Nitsche CJ, Jamieson N, Lerch MM, Mayerle JV. Drug induced pancreatitis. *Best Pract Res Clin Gastroenterol* 2010;24:143–155

18. Johnson DD, Palumbo PJ, Chu CP. Diabetic ketoacidosis in a community-based population. *Mayo Clin Proc* 1980;55:83–88

19. Wang ZH, Kihl-Selstam E, Eriksson JW. Ketoacidosis occurs in both type 1 and type 2 diabetes—a population-based study from northern Sweden. *Diabet Med* 2008;25:867–870

20. Centers for Disease Control. Age-adjusted percentage of adults aged 18 years or older with diagnosed diabetes who have hypertension, United States, 1995–2009. Available from http://www.cdc.gov/diabetes/statistics/comp/fig8.htm. Accessed 23 January 2015

3

Glucocorticoid, Mineralocorticoid, and Immunomodulatory Agents

GLUCOCORTICOID STEROIDS

In people with diabetes, systemic glucocorticoid steroid therapy impairs glycemic control via multiple mechanisms. Glucocorticoids induce insulin resistance, inhibit peripheral glucose utilization, stimulate lipolysis, and increase hepatic glucose production.[1-3] In addition, these steroids inhibit insulin secretion and insulin biosynthesis, stimulate glucagon release, and induce endoplasmic reticulum stress and β-cell apoptosis following prolonged exposure (Figure 3.1).[2,4-6] In people with prediabetes and those at high risk for type 2 diabetes (T2D), prolonged steroid therapy could worsen glucose tolerance and induce diabetes. There is significant heterogeneity in individual susceptibility to glucocorticoid-induced dysglycemia. Accurate data on the exact magnitude of risk are lacking, and the tendency to report mostly fasting glucose levels might mask the true prevalence of the problem.

Figure 3.1—Constellation of the diabetogenic actions of glucocorticoids. ER, endoplasmic reticulum.

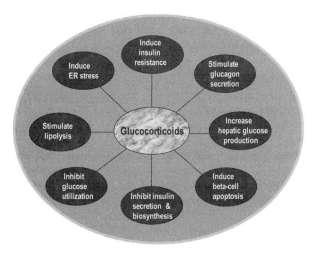

In one nested case control study based on a family practice database, the adjusted odds ratio for diabetes associated with three or more oral glucocorticoid prescriptions was 1.36 (95% confidence interval [CI] 1.10–1.69; P = 0.005).[7] Thus, the risk of treatment-emergent diabetes was increased by 36% following oral steroid exposure.[7] The diabetes risk is dependent on the dose and duration of glucocorticoid therapy, but even single doses of potent agents, such as dexamethasone, can induce transient hyperglycemia.[8] Genetic factors play a prominent role in determining susceptibility: in one study, a family history of diabetes increased the risk of steroid-induced diabetes tenfold.[9] Other risk factors for steroid-induced diabetes include the potency of steroid preparation, age, weight, decreased β-cell capacity, and a history of gestational diabetes (Table 3.1).[10,11] Compared with systemic therapy, inhaled or topical glucocorticoids or glucocorticoid eye drops have not been consistently associated with hyperglycemia.[6,7,12]

Table 3.1 — Risk Factors for Steroid-Induced Diabetes

■ Family history of diabetes

■ Type, dose, and duration of steroid therapy

■ History of gestational diabetes

■ Overweight or obesity

■ Older age

■ Decreased insulin secretory capacity

High doses of topical steroids, however, can sometimes induce hyperglycemia.[10] Reports are conflicting on the effects of intra-articular steroid injection on blood glucose levels.[13–15] Overall, the reported glucose excursions tend to be transient, returning to baseline within a few hours to 5 days following the injection of steroids into inflamed joints.[15,16]

Approach to Risk Reduction

When systemic glucocorticoid therapy is unavoidable, as in patients with acute severe asthma or transplant recipients, blood glucose levels should be monitored frequently and the antidiabetic regimen should be optimized. Insulin sensitizer drugs and insulin augmentation, alone or in combination, can help restore glycemic control in most patients with steroid-induced diabetes.[17] Because the metabolic effects of glucocorticoids are dose related, use of the minimum effective dose for treatment of the primary condition is recommended. For people with prediabetes and those at high risk for T2D, lifestyle modification (Table 3.2) has been shown to be effective in preventing diabetes and should be advocated empirically, although there are no specific data for the steroid-treated population. In experimental animals, treatment with etomoxir (an inhibitor of fatty acid oxidation) improves insulin sensitivity and reverses glucocorticoid-induced insulin resistance.[18]

Table 3.2—Approach to Prevention of Glucocorticoid-Induced Diabetes

- Identify risk factors for diabetes (age, family history, overweight/obesity, etc.)
- Monitor blood glucose frequently in high-risk subjects
- Recommend lifestyle modification for high-risk people
- Use minimum effective dose of glucocorticoid steroid
- Consider alternate-day regimen, if feasible
- Consider metformin for people with prediabetes (impaired fasting glucose and impaired glucose tolerance)

The possible prophylactic use of insulin sensitizers (e.g., thiazolidinediones [TZDs] and metformin) to prevent diabetes during prolonged steroid therapy is somewhat appealing.[19] Such an approach, however, would be an off-label use of metformin and TZDs; additionally, the judicious selection of appropriate candidates for such an intervention requires an exact treatment-emergent diabetes risk prediction capability that currently is elusive. Absent data from randomized controlled trials, the efficacy of prophylactic antidiabetes therapy is unknown, as are the number needed to treat, and the merit of such an approach over that of careful monitoring and lifestyle modification. On the basis of the aggregation of diabetes risk factors, underlying ailments, and the glucocorticoid regimen, patients deemed to be at particularly high risk for steroid-induced diabetes (Table 3.1) may be considered for training in ambulatory self–blood glucose monitoring. The training should include instructions on the expected range of fasting and nonfasting blood glucose values, and out-of-range values that should trigger contact with the treating physician. The record of home blood glucose measurement should be reviewed during clinic visits, to determine whether a pattern of dysglycemia is discernible. As a pragmatic compromise, metformin can be considered in addition to lifestyle modification in high-risk patients who show evidence of prediabetes (impaired glucose tolerance [IGT] and impaired fasting glucose [IFG]) before or during prolonged steroid therapy, to prevent progression to diabetes.[20]

The mechanism of action of glucocorticoids involves binding to the intracellular glucocorticoid receptor and subsequent interaction with nuclear targets. At the genomic level, the anti-inflammatory actions of glucocorticoids are mediated by transrepression of target genes, whereas the metabolic effects are mediated mostly by transactivation of genes. Thus, novel compounds in development (selective glucocorticoid receptor agonists [SEGRAs]) might be successful in selectively targeting inflammation, while avoiding adverse metabolic effects of glucocorticoids.[21] The future availability of SEGRAs would be a great advance in the prevention of glucocorticoid-induced diabetes.[22]

Although there are individual variations of therapeutic needs and response patterns, patients who develop hyperglycemia during treatment with gluco-corticoids frequently require insulin therapy for optimal glycemic control.[23] A detailed discussion of the management of breakthrough hyperglycemia during glucocorticoid therapy is beyond the scope of this work. Flexibility is required, however, so that the intensity of insulin treatment can be governed by the ambient glucocorticoid regimen, including consideration of the pharmacodynamics of the specific glucocorticoid in use. Some effective insulin regimens for control of steroid-induced diabetes in hospitalized patients are available.[24,25]

MINERALOCORTICOIDS: ALDOSTERONE AND GLUCOREGULATION

In his pioneering studies that described the syndrome of hyperaldosteronism in the 1950s, Dr. Conn observed an increased risk of diabetes in affected patients.[26] Although not fully understood, the mechanisms linking hyperaldosteronism to glucose intolerance and diabetes include hypokalemia, activation of reactive oxygen species and inflammatory cytokines, and impaired insulin secretion.[4,27,28] Hypokalemia induced by aldosterone activation of the mineralocorticoid receptor was once thought to be the dominant mechanism for dysglycemia through its negative effect on insulin secretion. Potassium repletion only partially restores insulin secretion and glucose tolerance, however. To explain the latter finding, direct inhibitory effects of aldosterone on glucose-stimulated insulin secretion have been observed in isolated pancreatic islets cells, probably through activation of reactive oxygen species.[28] Similar inhibitory effects of aldosterone on insulin signaling have been demonstrated in adipocytes and skeletal muscle cells. Thus, multiple mechanisms (including hypokalemia, mineralocorticoid receptor–mediated activation of reactive oxygen species and proinflammatory cytokines, insulin resistance, and impaired insulin secretion) link hyperaldosteronism to glucose intolerance and hyperglycemia. Interestingly, mineralocorticoid receptor blockade improves pancreatic insulin release, insulin-mediated glucose utilization, and endothelium-dependent vasorelaxation, all of which should ameliorate the deleterious effects of aldosterone on glucoregulation.[27]

The mineralocorticoid agent, fludrocortisone (Florinef), is prescribed widely for patients with primary adrenal insufficiency and conditions associated with aldosterone deficiency, hyperkalemia, orthostatic hypotension, and type IV renal tubular acidosis. To date, the clinical use of Florinef has not been associated with diabetes risk in published reports. As noted, mineralocorticoid antagonists, spironolactone and eplerenone, have been associated with improved insulin sensitivity and insulin secretion.[27]

IMMUNOMODULATORY AGENTS

Calcineurin Inhibitors and Post-Transplant Diabetes

Organ transplantation is an expanding area of modern medical practice, and diabetes is being increasingly diagnosed in organ recipients. Post-transplant diabetes (also known as new-onset diabetes after transplantation [NODAT]) refers to the occurrence of diabetes in subjects who previously did not have diabetes following transplantation. The development of NODAT is associated with adverse clinical outcomes, including renal allograft loss, post-transplant infections, cardiovascular disease, and increased mortality.[29-31] Variable incidence rates of NODAT have been reported over variable intervals among recipients of different organ transplants. The estimated rates of NODAT at 12 months or longer post-transplant are ~20% for kidney transplants, 9% to 21% for liver transplants, and ~20% for lung transplants.[32-34] Most of the data in this field are derived from analysis of renal transplants, because information on other types of transplants is limited. The peak incidence of NODAT appears to occur around 3 months post-transplant, but the risk of diabetes persists for much longer.

The clinical presentation of NODAT is consistent with T2D, and studies have identified insulin resistance and impaired β-cell function as the underlying mechanisms.[35] The insulin resistance can be induced in subjects who previously were normoglycemic and can be aggravated in subjects who have prediabetes, following organ transplantation. Medications used for post-transplant immunosuppression have been implicated in the pathogenesis of NODAT. The calcineurin inhibitors (tacrolimus and cyclosporine) and steroids have been the most documented drugs associated with the induction of NODAT. The agents, however, also are the most widely used immunosuppressive agents in the transplant population, and many other risk factors appear to influence the development of NODAT (Table 3.3).[32,36]

Table 3.3—Risk Factors for Post-Transplant Diabetes Mellitus

Nonmodifiable	Modifiable
Age >45 years	• Immunosuppressive regimen
Race	- Tacrolimus
	- Glucocorticoid steroids
Ethnicity	- Combined tacrolimus and steroid
	• Acute rejection
	• Prediabetes (impaired fasting glucose or impaired glucose tolerance)
	• Body mass (BMI > 25 kg/m²)
	• Cadaveric organ
	• Hepatitis-C infection

The mechanisms for steroid-induced insulin resistance are well known and were discussed in the preceding section. In contrast, the mechanisms whereby calcineurin inhibitors induce insulin resistance are not known precisely; however, calcineurin inhibitors have been reported to inhibit insulin gene transcription and decrease insulin secretion by the β-cells.[37] The reported ~20% incidence of NODAT for kidney transplant recipients at 1 year means that ~80% of graft recipients can expect to be free from diabetes.[32-34] Thus, immunosuppressive agents induce NODAT in a substantial minority of post-transplant patients, whereas a sizeable majority of such patients escape the diabetes risk, which underscores the contributory roles of other risk factors (Table 3.3). Notably, the risk of NODAT does not appear to be a class effect for the calcineurin inhibitors: in one study, treatment with tacrolimus was associated with a twofold higher incidence of NODAT (16.8% vs. 8.9%) than cyclosporine.[38] Prediabetes events also were more frequent with tacrolimus.

Approach to Management and Risk Reduction

The high prevalence of NODAT provides ample opportunity for developing evidence-based strategies for diabetes prevention, yet randomized controlled studies are scant.[39, 40] Pre-transplant lifestyle counseling would be most appropriate for high-risk patients, including those who are overweight or obese, and people with a family history of T2D (Tables 1.1 and 3.3). A screening fasting plasma glucose level or oral glucose tolerance test would help identify subjects with prediabetes (IFG or IGT) during the pre-transplant period, so that diabetes prevention counseling could be better targeted (Table 3.4). The goal of glycemic control in patients with NODAT is similar to the target (A1C <7%) for patients with diabetes in the general populace. For kidney transplant recipients, it is imperative to maintain excellent glycemic control, to protect the allograft from the risk of damage from diabetic nephropathy.

Table 3.4—Approach to Prevention of Post-Transplant Diabetes

Pre-Transplant Period

■ Document baseline fasting plasma glucose

■ Identify high-risk subjects

■ Initiate lifestyle intervention, including dietary and exercise counseling

Post-Transplant Period

■ Immunosuppressive regimen

■ Minimize steroid dose

Blood glucose monitoring, diabetes self-management education, dietary counseling, physical activity, and selective use of antidiabetic medications, constitute the basis of comprehensive diabetes management.[41-43] The mnemonic MEDEM (monitoring, education, diet, exercise, medication) can be used to recall the key elements of diabetes care. Depending on the organ transplanted and the state of renal, hepatic, and cardiac function, certain oral antidiabetic medications may be contraindicated in a given patient with NODAT, and insulin often is the drug of choice. In NODAT patients with intact renal, hepatic, and cardiac function, use of insulin sensitizers (metformin and TZDs) alone or in combination with secretagogues (sulfonylureas, glinides [repaglinide, nateglinide], gliptins [sitagliptin, saxagliptin, linagliptin, alogliption]) may be tried before proceeding to insulin. The α-glucosidase inhibitors (acarbose, miglitol), which act predominantly within the intestinal lumen to improve glycemic control, may be a consideration in cases in which systemic toxicity from other drugs needs to be avoided.

The management of NODAT should be undertaken in collaboration with the transplant team; whenever feasible, the lowest effective daily or alternate-day dose of steroid should be used to minimize the risk and magnitude of steroid-induced dysglycemia. Routine withdrawal or substitution of otherwise effective antirejection immunosuppressive therapy, solely because of NODAT, is ill-advised and could jeopardize the survival of the allograft. Nonetheless, small studies have suggested that substitution of tacrolimus with cyclosporine may be associated with improved glycemic control, and even resolution of NODAT in a few patients.[44,45] Because tacrolimus inhibits insulin secretion more potently (and is associated with higher risk for NODAT) than cyclosporine;[46,47] preferential use of cyclosporine would seem a judicious approach to diabetes risk reduction, provided, of course, that it is as effective as tacrolimus in organ protection. This is a complex risk-benefit calculation that has been well discussed by Chadban.[33]

Tumor Necrosis Factor-α Inhibitors

Tumor necrosis factor (TNF)-α is a proinflammatory cytokine that has been implicated in the etiology of a myriad of immunological disorders, including rheumatoid arthritis, Crohn's disease, psoriasis, and refractory asthma. Since the late 1990s, several monoclonal antibodies and fusion proteins, that inhibit TNF-α by blocking its receptor, have been introduced to clinical practice. These agents, collectively known as TNF-α inhibitors, include adalimumab, certolizumab pegol, etanercept, golimumab, and infliximab, and increasingly they are being prescribed for autoimmune disorders. Case reports have indicated that exposure to TNF-α inhibitors might improve glycemic control or even induce hypoglycemia in people with diabetes.[48–52] TNF-α induces pancreatic β-cell apoptosis and has been linked to insulin resistance and diabetes.[53,54] Thus, inhibition of TNF-α conceivably could improve glucose tolerance in subjects with diabetes. The likely mechanisms for such improvement include amelioration of insulin resistance[48,55] and preservation of β-cell function.[56] Given the increased prevalence of diabetes in patients with the autoimmune disorders,[57,58] close blood glucose monitoring and adjustment of antidiabetic regimen (as necessary) is advisable in patients receiving TNF-α inhibitors.

Interleukin-1 Receptor Antagonist

Interleukin (IL)-1 is overexpressed in pancreatic β-cells of patients with T2D and is known to impair insulin secretion and induce β-cell apoptosis.[59,60] Because progressive β-cell dysfunction underlies the pathophysiology of T2D, interventions that ameliorate β-cell apoptosis can be expected to decrease diabetes risk. In recent randomized placebo-controlled trials, short-term treatment with anakinra (100 mg QD subcutaneously for 13 weeks), a recombinant human IL-1 receptor antagonist, was shown to reduce inflammatory markers, improve β-cell function, and improve glycemic control in patients with T2D.[61,62] The improvement in β-cell function was demonstrable 39 weeks after the last dose of anakinra,[62] which suggests a cellular rather than humoral mechanism and raises hope for IL-1 inhibition as a future strategy for diabetes prevention.

Interferons

The interferons (IFNs) belong to a cytokine family of regulatory peptides that exhibit antiviral, antiproliferative, and immunomodulatory properties.[63] Advances in basic and translational research have led to clinical applications of some members of the IFN family in the treatment of viral infections and certain malignancies. For example, IFN-α is well established as an effective treatment for hepatitis C infection. Following its wide clinical use, reports of diabetes or dysglycemia in patients treated with IFN-α have appeared.[64,65] The cellular effects associated with IFNs include destruction of pancreatic islet cells (via an autoimmune mechanism) and possibly induction of insulin resistance at the postreceptor level.[66-68]

The incidence of treatment-emergent diabetes in patients receiving chronic IFN treatment for hepatitis C infection appears modest. In one report, 7 out of 202 (3.4%) patients developed diabetes and 33 (16.3%) developed prediabetes (IFG) during 5–16 years (median 8 years) of chronic IFN-α therapy.[69] The diabetes associated with IFN therapy often requires treatment with insulin; the insulin requirement may be transient or permanent. The fact that patients with hepatitis C infection have an increased risk for diabetes (independent of treatment) complicates the interpretation of reports of IFN-associated diabetes in such patients.[70,71] Rarely, patients receiving pegylated IFN therapy for hepatitis C have presented with diabetic ketoacidosis (curiously in conjunction with hyperthyroidism).[72]

REFERENCES

1. Fain JN. Effects of dexamethasone and 2-deoxy-D-glucose on fructose and glucose metabolism by incubated adipose tissue. *J Biol Chem* 1964;239:958–962

2. Chan JC, Cockram CS. Drug-induced disturbances of carbohydrate metabolism. *Adverse Drug React Toxicol Rev* 1991;10:1–29

3. Andrews RC, Herlihy O, Livingstone DE, Andrew R, Walker BR. Abnormal cortisol metabolism and tissue sensitivity to cortisol in patients with glucose intolerance. *J Clin Endocrinol Metab* 2002;87:5587–5593

4. Fallo F, Veglio F, Bertello C, et al. Prevalence and characteristics of the metabolic syndrome in primary aldosteronism. *J Clin Endocrinol Metab* 2006;91:454–459

5. Ranta F, Avram D, Berchtold S, et al. Dexamethasone induces cell death in insulin-secreting cells, an effect reversed by exendin-4. *Diabetes* 2006;55:1380–1390

6. van Raalte DH, Diamant M. Steroid diabetes: from mechanism to treatment? *Neth J Med* 2014;72:62–72

7. Gulliford MC, Charlton J, Latinovic R. Risk of diabetes associated with prescribed glucocorticoids in a large population. *Diabetes Care* 2006;29:2728–2729

8. Dagogo-Jack S, Selke G, Melson AK, Newcomer JW. Robust leptin secretory responses to dexamethasone in obese subjects. *J Clin Endocrinol Metab* 1997;82:3230–3233

9. Fajans SS, Conn JW. An approach to the prediction of diabetes mellitus by modification of the glucose tolerance test with cortisone. *Diabetes* 1954;3:296–302

10. Heazell AE, Shina A, Bhatti NR. A case of gestational diabetes arising following treatment with glucocorticoids for pemphigoid gestations. *J Maternal-Fetal Neonatal Med* 2005;18:353–355

11. McCullen MK, Ahmed I. Drug-induced hyperglycemia and diabetes mellitus. In: *Type 2 Diabetes, Principles and Practice*. 2nd ed. Goldstein BJ and Müller-Wieland D, Eds. Taylor & Francis, New York, 2007, p. 513–528

12. Blackburn D, Hux J, Mamdani M. Quantification of the risk of corticosteroid-induced diabetes mellitus among the elderly. *J Gen Intern Med* 2002;17:717–720

13. Black DM, Filak AT. Hyperglycemia with non-insulin-dependent diabetes following intraarticular steroid injection. *J Fam Pract* 1989;28:462–463

14. Habib GS, Abu-Ahmad R. Lack of effect of corticosteroid injection at the shoulder joint on blood glucose levels in diabetic patients. *Clin Rheumatol* 2007;26:566–568

15. Habib GS, Bashir M, Jabbour A. Increased blood glucose levels following intra-articular injection of methylprednisolone acetate in patients with controlled diabetes and symptomatic osteoarthritis of the knee. *Ann Rheum Dis* 2008;67:1790–1791

16. Habib G, Khazin F, Chernin M. Continuous blood glucose monitoring in a patient with type 2 diabetes who underwent intraarticular betamethasone injection for knee osteoarthritis. *Arthritis Rheumatol* 2014;66:230; doi: 10.1002/art.38209

17. Brady VJ, Grimes D, Armstrong T, LoBiondo-Wood G. Management of steroid-induced hyperglycemia in hospitalized patients with cancer: a review. *Oncol Nurs Forum* 2014;41:E355–365

18. Guillaume-Gentil C, Assimacopoulos-Jeannet F, Jeanrenaud B. Involvement of non-esterified fatty acid oxidation in glucocorticoid-induced peripheral insulin resistance in vivo in rats. *Diabetologia* 1993;36:899–906

19. Willi SM, Kennedy A, Brant BP, Wallace P, Rogers NL, Garvey WT. Effective use of thiazolidinediones for the treatment of glucocorticoid-induced diabetes. *Diabetes Res Clin Pract* 2002;58:87–96

20. Nathan DM, Davidson MB, DeFronzo RA, et al. Impaired fasting glucose and impaired glucose tolerance: implications for care. *Diabetes Care* 2007;30:753–759

21. Schacke H, Berger M, Rehwinkel H, Asadullah K. Selective glucocorticoid receptor agonists (SEGRAs): novel ligands with an improved therapeutic index. *Mol Cell Endocrinol* 2007;275:109–117

22. van Lierop MJ, Alkema W, Laskewitz AJ, et al. Org 214007-0: a novel nonsteroidal selective glucocorticoid receptor modulator with full anti-inflammatory properties and improved therapeutic index. *PLoS One* 2012;7:e48385

23. Baldwin D, Apel J. Management of hyperglycemia in hospitalized patients with renal insufficiency or steroid-induced diabetes. *Curr Diab Rep* 2013;13:114–120

24. Grommesh B, Lausch MJ, Vannelli AJ, et al. Hospital insulin protocol aims for glucose control in glucocorticoid-induced hyperglycemia. *Endocr Pract* 22 Oct 2015 [Epub ahead of print]

25. Ruiz de Adana MS, Colomo N, Maldonado-Araque C, et al. Randomized clinical trial of the efficacy and safety of insulin glargine vs. NPH insulin as basal insulin for the treatment of glucocorticoid induced hyperglycemia using continuous glucose monitoring in hospitalized patients with type 2 diabetes and respiratory disease. *Diabetes Res Clin Pract.* 20 Sep 2015 [Epub ahead of print]

26. Conn JW. Presidential address. I. Painting background. II. Primary aldosteronism, a new clinical syndrome. *J Lab Clin Med* 1955;45:3–17

27. Sowers JR, Whaley-Connell A, Epstein M. Narrative review: the emerging clinical implications of the role of aldosterone in the metabolic syndrome and resistant hypertension. *Ann Intern Med* 2009;150:776–783

28. Luther JM. Effects of aldosterone on insulin sensitivity and secretion. *Steroids* 2014;91:54–60

29. Cosio FG, Pesavento TE, Kim S, et al. Patient survival after renal transplantation: IV. Impact of post-transplant diabetes. *Kidney Int* 2002;62:1440–1446

30. Chapman JR, O'Connell PJ, Nankivell BJ. Chronic renal allograft dysfunction. *J Am Soc Nephrol* 2005;16:3015–3026

31. Hjelmesaeth J, Hartmann A, Leivestad T, Holdaas H, Sagedal S, Olstad M, Jenssen T. The impact of early diagnosed new-onset post-transplantation diabetes mellitus on survival and major cardiac events. *Kidney Int* 2006;69:588–595

32. Kasiske B, Snyder JJ, Gilbertson D, et al. Diabetes mellitus after kidney transplantation in the United States. *Am J Transplant* 2003;3:178–185

33. Chadban S. New-onset diabetes after transplantation—should it be a factor in choosing an immunosuppressant regimen for kidney transplant recipients. *Nephrol Dial Transplant* 2008;23:1816–1818

34. Bonato V, Cataldo D, Dotta F, Carmellini M. Diagnosis and approach to posttransplant diabetes. *Curr Diab Rep* 2009;9:317–323

35. Hjelmesaeth J, Midtvedt K, Jenssen T, et al. Insulin resistance after renal transplantation: impact of immunosuppressive and antihypertensive therapy. *Diabetes Care* 2001;24:2121–2126

36. Vesco L, Busson M, Bedrossian J, et al. Diabetes mellitus after renal transplantation: characteristics, outcomes, and risk factors. *Transplantation* 1996;61:1475–1478

37. Oetjen E, Baun D, Beimesche S, et al. Inhibition of human insulin gene transcription by the immunosuppressive drugs cyclosporine and tacrolimus in primary, mature islets of transgenicmice. *Mol Pharmacol* 2003;63:1289–1295

38. Vincenti F, Friman S, Scheuermann E, et al. Results of an international, randomized trial comparing glucose metabolism disorders and outcome with cyclosporine versus tacrolimus. *Am J Transplant* 2007;7:1506–1514

39. Lane JT, Dagogo-Jack S. Approach to the patient with new-onset diabetes after transplant (NODAT). *J Clin Endocrinol Metab* 2011;96:3289–3297

40. Gosmanov AR, Dagogo-Jack S. Predicting, managing and preventing new-onset diabetes after transplantation. *Minerva Endocrinol* 2012;37:233–246

41. Haas L, Maryniuk M, Beck J, et al.; 2012 Standards Revision Task Force. National standards for diabetes self-management education and support. *Diabetes Care* 2012;35:2393–2401

42. Powers MA, Bardsley J, Cypress M, et al. Diabetes self-management education and support in type 2 diabetes: a joint position statement of the American Diabetes Association, the American Association of Diabetes Educators, and the Academy of Nutrition and Dietetics. *Diabetes Educ* 2015;41:417–430

43. American Diabetes Association. Standards of medical care in diabetes—2015. *Diabetes Care* 2015;38(Suppl. 1):S5–S87

44. Dumortier J, Bernard S, Bouffard Y, et al. Conversion from tacrolimus to cyclosporine in liver transplanted patients with diabetes mellitus. *Liver Transpl* 2006;12:659–664

45. Ghisdal L, Bouchta NB, Broeders N, et al. Conversion from tacrolimus to cyclosporine a for new-onset diabetes after transplantation: a single centre experience in renal transplanted patients and review of the literature. *Transpl Int* 2008;21:146–151

46. Redmon JB, Olson LK, Armstrong MB, et al. Effects of tacrolimus (FK506) on human insulin gene expression, insulin mRNA levels, and insulin secretion in HIT-T15 cells. *J Clin Invest* 1996;98:2786–2793

47. Webster AC, Woodroffe RC, Taylor RS, Chapman JR, Craig JC. Tacrolimus versus ciclosporin as primary immunosuppression for kidney transplant recipients: meta-analysis and meta-regression of randomised trial data. *BMJ* 2005;331:810, Epub 2005 Sept 12

48. Kiortsis DN, Mavridis AK, Vasakos S, Nikas SN, Drosos AA. Effects of infliximab treatment on insulin resistance in patients with rheumatoid arthritis and ankylosing spondylitis. *Ann Rheumatic Dis* 2005;64:765–766

49. van Eijk IC, Peters MJ, Nurmohamed MT, van Deutekom AW, Dijkmans BA, Simsek S. Decrease of fructosamine levels during treatment with adalimumab in patients with both diabetes and rheumatoid arthritis. *Eur J Endocrinol* 2007;156:291–293

50. Wambier CG, Foss-Freitas MC, Paschoal RS, et al. Severe hypoglycemia after initiation of anti-tumor necrosis factor therapy with etanercept in a patient with generalized pustular psoriasis and type 2 diabetes mellitus. *J Am Acad Dermatol* 2009;60:883–885

51. Cheung D, Bryer-Ash M. Persistent hypoglycemia in a patient with diabetes taking etanercept for the treatment of psoriasis. *J Am Acad Dermatol* 2009;60:1032–1036

52. Czajkowska JB, Shutty B, Zito S. Development of low blood glucose readings in nine non-diabetic patients treated with tumor necrosis factor-alpha inhibitors: a case series. *J Med Case Rep* 2012;6:5. doi: 10.1186/1752-1947-6-5

53. Zinman B, Hanley AJ, Harris SB, et al. Circulating tumor necrosis factor-alpha concentrations in a native Canadian population with high rates of type 2 diabetes mellitus. *J Clin Endocrinol Metab* 1999;84:27–28

54. Obayashi H, Hasegawa G, Fukui M, et al. Tumor necrosis factor microsatellite polymorphism influences the development of insulin dependency in adult-onset diabetes patients with the DRB1*1502-DQB1*0601 allele and anti-glutamic acid decarboxylase antibodies. *J Clin Endocrinol Metab* 2000;85:3348–3351

55. Martínez-Abundis E, Reynoso-von Drateln C, Hernández-Salazar E, González-Ortiz M. Effect of etanercept on insulin secretion and insulin sensitivity in a randomized trial with psoriatic patients at risk for developing type 2 diabetes mellitus. *Arch Dermatol Res* 2007;299:461–465

56. Mastrandrea L, Yu J, Behrens T, Buchlis J, Albini C, Fourtner S, Quattrin T. Etanercept treatment in children with new-onset type 1 diabetes: pilot randomized, placebo-controlled, double-blind study. *Diabetes Care* 2009;32:1244–1249

57. Brauchli YB, Jick SS, Meier CR. Psoriasis and the risk of incident diabetes mellitus: a population-based study. *Br J Dermatol* 2008;159:1331–1337

58. Cohen AD, Sherf M, Vidavsky L, Vardy DA, Shapiro J, Meyerovitch J. Association between psoriasis and the metabolic syndrome. A cross-sectional study. *Dermatology* 2008;216:152–155

59. Bendtzen K, Mandrup-Poulsen T, Nerup J, Nielsen JH, Dinarello CA, Svenson M. Cytotoxicity of human pI 7 interleukin-1 for pancreatic islets of Langerhans. *Science* 1986;232:1545–1547

60. Maedler K, Sergeev P, Ris F, et al. Glucose-induced β cell production of IL-1β contributes to glucotoxicity in human pancreatic islets. *J Clin Invest* 2002;110:851–860

61. Larsen CM, Faulenbach M, Vaag A, et al. Interleukin-1-receptor antagonist in type 2 diabetes mellitus. *N Engl J Med* 2007;356:1517–1526

62. Larsen CM, Faulenbach M, Vaag A, Ehses JA, Donath MY, Mandrup-Poulsen T. Sustained effects of interleukin-1 receptor antagonist treatment in type 2 diabetes. *Diabetes Care* 2009;32:1663–1668

63. Dagogo-Jack S. Peptide regulatory factors: physiological and clinical implications. *Niger Med J* 1991;21:144–149

64. Fabris P, Betterle C, Greggio NA, et al. Insulin-dependent diabetes mellitus during alpha interferon therapy for chronic viral hepatitis. *J Hepatol* 1998;28:514–517

65. Chedin P, Cahen-Varsaux J, Boyer N. Non-insulin dependent diabetes mellitus development during interferon alpha therapy for chronic viral hepatitis. *Ann Intern Med* 1996;125:521

66. Foulis AK, Farquharson MA, Meager A. Immunoreactive alpha-interferon in insulin secreting beta-cells in type 1 diabetes mellitus. *Lancet* 1987;2:1423–1427

67. Pankewycz OG, Guan J-X, Benedict JF. Cytokines as mediators of autoimmune diabetes and diabetic complications. *Endocrine Rev* 1995;16:164–171

68. Konrad T, Zeuzem S, Vicini P, et al. Evaluation of factors controlling glucose tolerance in patients with HCV infection before and after 4 months therapy with interferon-alpha. *Eur J Clin Invest* 2000;30:111–121

69. Giordanino C, Bugianesi E, Smedile A, et al. Incidence of type 2 diabetes mellitus and glucose abnormalities in patients with chronic hepatitis C infection by response to treatment: results of a cohort study. *Am J Gastroenterol* 2008;103:2481–2487

70. Ozylikau E, Arslan M. Increased prevalence of diabetes mellitus in patients with chronic hepatitis C virus infection. *Am J Gastroenterol* 1997;91:1480–1481

71. Huang JF, Yu ML, Dai CY, et al. Reappraisal of the characteristics of glucose abnormalities in patients with chronic hepatitis C infection. *Am J Gastroenterol* 2008;103:1933–1940

72. Soultati AS, Dourakis SP, Alexopoulou A, Deutsch M, Archimandritis AJ. Simultaneous development of diabetic ketoacidosis and Hashitoxicosis in a patient treated with pegylated interferon-alpha for chronic hepatitis C. *World J Gastroenterol* 2007;13:1292–1294

4

Sex Steroids and Gonadotropin-Releasing Hormone Analogs

ESTROGENS AND PROGESTINS

Some cross-sectional studies have reported an association between higher plasma levels of estradiol and increased risk of type 2 diabetes (T2D) in men and women.[1] The association of estradiol levels with increased risk of T2D remained after controlling for BMI.[1] A report from the prospective Diabetes Prevention Program (DPP) showed that plasma levels of estrone sulfate were directly associated with 2-h postload oral glucose tolerance test (OGTT) plasma glucose levels in men and premenopausal women.[2] Among DPP male participants, diabetes risk was directly associated with estrone (hazard ratio [HR] 1.101 [95% CI 1.059–1.145]), estrone sulfate (HR 1.003 [95% CI 1.001–1.005]), and estradiol (HR 1.130 [95% CI 10.45–1.221]). The associations with estrogens persisted after adjustment for waist circumference, insulin resistance, and β-cell function.[2]

Remarkably, circulating estrogens were not associated with diabetes outcomes in women, despite being correlated with 2-h postload OGTT plasma glucose values.[2] Thus, the available data from cross-sectional and prospective studies indicate that higher levels of endogenous estrogens are associated with increased risk of T2D, with perhaps a stronger association in men. Because men rarely receive treatment with estrogens, the clinical implications for men of the aforementioned studies for diabetes risk in women may be modest.

Oral Contraceptives and Estrogen Replacement

Studies linking oral contraceptives (OCs) to diabetes risk have been conflicting, and the findings depend somewhat on the composition of OCs and whether women were tested in the basal (fasting) state or following glucose challenge in an OGTT. Depending on the dose and formulation, mild to moderate fluctuations in blood glucose can occur following initiation of OC therapy, although the clinical significance of such fluctuations is unclear.[3] A cross-sectional study of fasting glucose, insulin, C-peptide, and HbA$_{1c}$ levels among women who had never used OCs, current users of OCs, and former users of OCs in the Third National Health and Nutrition Examination Survey (NHANES 1988–1994)[4] concluded that current users of OCs did not have elevated values for any of the four measures of glucose metabolism.[5]

In contrast to the NHANES 1988–1994 data based on fasting blood measurements, a study in which OGTTs were performed in 1,060 women taking OCs and 418 control women taking no OCs found different results. The index participants were taking one of nine types of OCs for at least 3 months. Two of the formulations were progestin-only agents and seven were combinations of progestin (150–1,000 µ) and ethinyl estradiol (30–40 µ). The authors found that combination OCs were associated with a worsening of glucose tolerance.[6] Compared with the women not exposed to contraceptives, women taking OCs had ~50% increase in the OGTT plasma glucose and ~30% increase in insulin and C-peptide levels, which indicates that exposure to OCs had induced insulin resistance.[6] In another report,[7] sixteen hyperandrogenic women tested before and 6 months after receiving desogestrel-containing OC showed deterioration of glucose tolerance (two of them developed diabetes).

Progestin-containing formulations are believed to be more liable to induce hyperglycemia, whereas low-dose triphasic OCs appear to be less so.[8,9] Reports are conflicting, however, regarding whether a dose–response relationship actually exists between progestins and glycemia.[6,10] In general, the OC-induced insulin resistance usually is mild and reversible; it is most likely a steroid effect, and it can be minimized by selecting preparations with low estrogen and progesterone content.

Estrogen replacement therapy in menopausal women has the same potential effects on carbohydrate metabolism. In practice, however, patients with diabetes on OCs or estrogen replacement therapy rarely develop significant perturbations in glycemic control.

Approach to Risk Reduction

Antidiabetic drug doses should be optimized in women with diabetes who experience blood glucose fluctuations during treatment with OCs.[11] Other women receiving OCs should be advised to undergo blood glucose testing if they develop symptoms suggestive of diabetes. The prevalence of OC-induced diabetes is unknown; the risk appears to be inconsistent, and causality has not been established. Therefore, diabetes (or the risk for diabetes) would not be a rational contraindication to the appropriate use of OCs. As the evidence suggests that insulin resistance from the steroidogenic effects of OCs might occur in some women following glucose challenge, lifestyle counseling for overweight or obese, high-risk women would be appropriate. Cigarette smoking and hypertension compound the adverse effect of OCs, so maintenance of optimal blood pressure is important, and counseling also should include smoking cessation.[12,13] Furthermore, use of low-dose triphasic formulations may be associated with less metabolic perturbations than higher dose OCs.[14]

ANDROGENS, SEX HORMONE BINDING GLOBULIN, AND GLUCOREGULATION

A state of *hypogonadotropic hypogonadism* has been described in some men with T2D.[15] Such men tend to have plasma free testosterone levels that fall below the normal range, serum levels of luteinizing hormone (LH) and follicle-stimulating hormone (FSH) that are not elevated (i.e., inappropriately normal), and a tendency to manifest features of insulin resistance. Some evidence suggests that supplemental testosterone therapy improves insulin sensitivity and metabolic endpoints in men with diabetes-related hypogonadotropic hypogonadism.[16–19] By contrast, other studies of testosterone replacement in men with T2D and hypogonadism showed no demonstrable benefit on glycemic control.[20,21] Cross-sectional studies in the general population have reported a correlation between circulating testosterone levels and insulin sensitivity, and some studies have also suggested a link between testosterone levels and the risk of T2D.[22] Ding et al.[1] performed a meta-analysis of data from 80 publications derived from 43 prospective and cross-sectional studies (total population 6,974 women and 6,427 men), and calculated the relative risks (RRs) of T2D in relation to testosterone levels in men and women. Using random effects and meta-regression analysis in the pooled sample, the cross-sectional studies showed that testosterone level was significantly lower in men with T2D (mean difference –76.6 ng/dL; 95% CI [–99.4 to –53.6] and significantly higher in women with T2D compared with controls (mean difference 6.1 ng/dL; 95% CI [2.3–10.1]. (Parenthetically, estradiol levels were significantly higher in men with T2D compared with controls.) The findings from prospective studies were concordant: men with higher testosterone levels (range, 449.6–605.2 ng/dL) had a 42% lower risk of T2D (RR 0.58; 95% CI [0.39–0.87]).[1] As in the cross-sectional studies, the findings in women were opposite: higher testosterone tended to be associated with increased risk of T2D.[1] These and other reports indicate that endogenous sex hormones may differentially modulate diabetes risk in the two sexes, such that high testosterone levels are associated with higher risk of T2D in women but with lower risk in men (Figure 4.1).[23–28] These relationships are somewhat attenuated but persist even

Figure 4.1—Circulating testosterone (T) and estradiol (E2) are bound to sex hormone binding globulin (SHBG). Cytosolic free T and E2 molecules access nuclear receptors and activate transcriptional machinery, leading to differential alteration of glucoregulation in men and women.

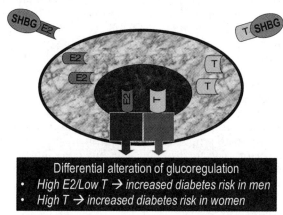

after adjustment for traditional diabetes risk factors, age, race, menopausal status, diabetes diagnosis criteria, BMI, and waist-to-hip ratio.[1]

Sex Hormone Binding Globulin

In the said meta-analysis by Ding et al.,[1] data on sex hormone binding globulin (SHBG) levels and diabetes status were available for 2,500 men and 4,765 women from 23 cross-sectional studies and 466 cases of diabetes from 10 prospective studies. In cross-sectional studies, both men and women with T2D had lower plasma levels of SHBG than did controls, although the difference reached significance only among women. In pooled data from the cross-sectional and prospective studies, women with circulating SHBG levels of ≥60 nmol/L (and therefore lower free testosterone levels) had an 80% lower risk of T2D compared with women whose SHBG levels were <60 nmol/L.[1] The latter finding is in agreement with observations linking SHBG, bioavailable testosterone, and estradiol with insulin resistance and glucose levels in men and women.[29–31] SHBG binds and transports both testosterone and estradiol: the binding affinity for testosterone is twice the binding for estradiol. Thus, the reported associations of SHBG with insulin resistance and glucose homeostasis could be mediated through differential modulation of bioavailable (free) testosterone and estradiol levels by SHBG in men and women. The exact mechanisms underlying the associations among SHBG, the individual sex steroids, glucoregulation, and diabetes risk are not completely understood, however.

Mather et al.[2] analyzed steroid sex hormones and SHBG levels in relation to glucose homeostasis and incident T2D in the multicenter Diabetes Prevention Program (DPP). The prospective DPP cohort was composed of 2,898 subjects with prediabetes, including 969 men, 948 premenopausal women not taking exogenous sex hormones, 550 postmenopausal women not taking exogenous sex hormones, and 431 postmenopausal women taking exogenous sex hormones. The DPP participants were randomized to receive intensive lifestyle intervention, metformin, or placebo. The specific analytical outcomes were associations of steroid sex hormones and SHBG with glycemia and incident diabetes over a median follow-up of 3.0 years. The findings showed that testosterone and dihydrotestosterone (DHT) levels were inversely associated with fasting glucose in men. SHBG was associated with fasting glucose in premenopausal women not taking exogenous sex hormones and in postmenopausal women on hormone replacement therapy. SHBG, however, was not associated with plasma glucose in men or in postmenopausal women not taking exogenous sex hormones.[2] Consistent with prior reports, diabetes incidence in the DPP cohort was inversely associated with testosterone and directly associated with estrone and estradiol levels in men. Notably, the association of diabetes with testosterone disappeared after adjustment for waist circumference. Sex steroids were not associated with diabetes outcomes in women, and SHBG levels and SHBG single-nucleotide polymorphisms did not predict incident diabetes in the DPP population.[2]

Testosterone and Anabolic Steroids for Diabetes Prevention

It must be stressed that epidemiological reports of an association between higher testosterone levels and decreased risk of T2D do not prove that testosterone is protective for T2D. Neither does the related finding of lower testosterone levels in men with T2D prove causality. Multiple mediators (including body composition and inflammatory cytokines) could be involved in any putative mechanisms linking diabetes risk and sex hormone levels. Some but not all intervention trials of testosterone augmentation in hypogonadal men with diabetes have shown favorable metabolic effects (decreased adiposity, improved insulin sensitivity, and suppression of inflammatory markers).[16,18–20] Those findings, however, cannot be validly extrapolated to support a role for testosterone supplementation in the primary prevention of diabetes.

Along the same lines, it has been speculated that the use of anabolic steroids possibly might be beneficial in reversing insulin resistance and the metabolic syndrome, thereby preventing overt diabetes.[32] Anabolic androgenic steroids, especially when used surreptitiously, have been associated with a broad range of toxic effects, including decreased levels of high-density lipoprotein cholesterol, polycythemia, testicular atrophy, gynecomastia, cardiovascular disease, peliosis hepatis, and hepatic neoplasia. Millions of men with systemic illnesses, overweight or obesity, or nonspecific deconditioning may have serum testosterone levels that fall below the lower reference. Also, serum testosterone levels decline as a function of age in men: typical average levels at age 60 years are ~40% lower, compared with levels in men ages 20–29 years.[33–38] Thus, testosterone levels below the normal range occur frequently in older men. It has been argued that poor health status, rather than aging, accounts for much of the decline in testosterone levels in older men.[39] Incidentally, the risk of T2D is increased in older, sedentary, and overweight or obese men, the same population in whom a coincidental finding of low testosterone can be expected. Notably, the effects of testosterone supplementation on diabetes incidence and other clinical endpoints have not been well studied in randomized, controlled trials.[38]

As no compelling studies have been conducted in the relevant at-risk population to inform such a strategy, the routine testing and treatment of men with low testosterone cannot be recommended as a means to preventing T2D. Long-term safety data on the prostatic, hematological, lipid, cardiovascular, and other clinical effects of therapy with testosterone or other androgen are lacking. Thus, the largely unknown long-term risks of androgen therapy in older men must be counterweighed against the questionable expectation that such treatment would improve glucoregulation and prevent diabetes.[40] In 2014, a U.S. Food and Drug Administration panel declared that, unlike pathologic hypogonadism, age-related decline in testosterone is not a recognized disease and that testosterone treatment for that indication is not of proven efficacy or safety.[41] Clearly, routine androgen replacement is unwarranted: a more rational and evidence-based approach to diabetes prevention should focus on lifestyle counseling, emphasizing healthy nutrition and increased physical activity.[42]

ANDROGEN-DEPRIVATION THERAPY WITH GONADOTROPIN-RELEASING HORMONE AGONISTS

As prostatic growth depends on dihydrotestosterone, an androgen metabolite, androgen-deprivation therapy has become standard treatment for prostate cancer. Nonsurgical androgen-deprivation is achieved using gonadotropin-releasing hormone (GnRH) agonists, such as Zoladex (goserelin), Lupron (leuprolide), Trelstar (triptorelin), Vantas (histrelin), and Synarel (nafarelin). GnRH agonists have been associated with increased risk for insulin resistance and hyperglycemia among men without a history of diabetes.[43-46] Emerging reports also suggest that androgen-deprivation therapy with GnRH agonists may worsen glycemic control among men with diabetes.[47] In a cohort study using a U.S. Veterans Administration (VA) database, HbA_{1c} levels and intensification of diabetes therapy were assessed among 2,237 men with prostate cancer and diabetes who were treated with GnRH agonists and a propensity-matched equal group of men with prostate cancer who were not treated with GnRH agonists. The changes in HbA_{1c} levels at baseline and at 1 and 2 years, and the time to intensification of diabetes treatment, were compared in the GnRH agonist-treated and control groups. The authors found that GnRH agonist treatment was associated with a significant increase in HbA_{1c} and a need for additional diabetes medication.[47]

Learned societies, including the American Heart Association, the American Urological Association, and the American Cancer Society, have issued advisory regarding possible increased risks of diabetes, myocardial infarction, stroke, and sudden death among men with prostate cancer receiving androgen deprivation therapy (ADT).[48] The FDA also has issued a warning regarding potential diabetes risk associated with GnRH agonists.[49] The potential mechanisms for an association between ADT and increased cardiometabolic risks include decreased lean mass,[50-52] increased fat mass,[45,53] increased insulin resistance,[54] and dyslipidemia together with a procoagulant state.[55]

The actual risk of GnRH agonist-induced diabetes is unknown but likely to be modest; in the VA database study, the absolute increase in HbA_{1c} attributable to GnRH treatment was ~0.2%.[47] Nonetheless, individual variability in the risk of diabetes can be expected, depending on family history, adiposity, and other factors. The FDA advisory recommends that patients receiving treatment with GnRH agonists should undergo periodic monitoring of blood glucose or HbA_{1c}. Health-care professionals also should monitor patients for signs and symptoms suggestive of cardiovascular disease and manage according to current clinical practice.[49] It seems prudent practice to perform screening for diabetes and cardiovascular risk factors in men with prostate cancer before initiation of ADT. Those with preexisting diabetes should be monitored closely during GnRH treatment and any exacerbation of hyperglycemia should be managed with intensification of antidiabetes regimen. People with evidence of prediabetes at baseline should receive lifestyle counseling, and close surveillance for possible worsening of dysglycemia following initiation of GnRH agonists. It is good practice to pay attention to comorbid risk factors, such as hypertension, dyslipidemia, and cigarette smoking.

REFERENCES

1. Ding EL, Song Y, Malik VS, Liu S. Sex differences of endogenous sex hormones and risk of type 2 diabetes: a systematic review and meta-analysis. *JAMA* 2006;295(11):1288–1299

2. Mather KJ, Kim C, Christophi CA, et al. Steroid sex hormones, sex hormone-binding globulin, and diabetes incidence in the Diabetes Prevention Program. *J Clin Endocrinol Metab* 2015;100:3778–3786

3. Gaspard UJ. Metabolic effects of oral contraceptives. *Am J Obstet Gynecol* 1987;157:1029–1041

4. Centers for Disease Control and Prevention. Third National Health and Nutrition Examination Survey (NHANES 1988–1994). http://www.cdc.gov/nchs/nhanes/nh3data.htm (accessed February 14, 2016)

5. Troisi RJ, Cowie CC, Harris MI. Oral contraceptive use and glucose metabolism in a national sample of women in the United States. *Am J Obstet Gynecol* 2000;183:389–395

6. Godsland IF, Crook D, Simpson R, et al. The effects of different formulations of oral contraceptive agents on lipid and carbohydrate metabolism. *N Eng J Med* 1990;323:1375–1381

7. Nader S, Riad-Gabriel MG, Saad MF. The effect of a desogestrel-containing oral contraceptive on glucose tolerance and leptin concentrations in hyperandrogenic women. *J Clin Endocrinol Metab* 1997;82:3074–3077

8. Xiang AH, Kawakubo M, Kjos SL, Buchanan TA. Long-acting injectable progestin contraception and risk of type 2 diabetes in Latino women with prior gestational diabetes. *Diabetes Care* 2006;29:613–617

9. Spellacy WN, Tsibris JC, Ellindson AB. Carbohydrate metabolic studies in women using a levonorgestrel/ethinyl estradiol containing triphasic oral contraceptive for eighteen months. *Int J Gynaecol Obstet* 1991;35:69–71

10. Rosenthal AD, Shu X, Jin F, et al. Oral contraceptive use and risk of diabetes among Chinese women. *Contraception* 2004;69:251–257

11. Shawe J, Lawrenson R. Hormonal contraception in women with diabetes mellitus: special consideration. *Treat Endocrinol* 2003;2:321–330

12. Godsland IF, Crook D, Devenport M, Wynn V. Relationships between blood pressure, oral contraceptive use and metabolic risk markers for cardiovascular disease. *Contraception* 1995;52:143–149

13. Suchon P, Al Frouh F, Henneuse A, et al. Risk factors for venous thromboembolism in women under combined oral contraceptive. The PILl Genetic Risk Monitoring (PILGRIM) Study. *Thromb Haemost* 20 Aug 2015 [Epub ahead of print]

14. Lachnit-Fixson U. The role of triphasic levonorgestrel in oral contraception: a review of metabolic and hemostatic effects. *Gynecol Endocrinol* 1996;10:207–218

15. Chandel A, Dhindsa S, Topiwala S, Chaudhuri A, Dandona P. Testosterone concentration in young patients with diabetes. *Diabetes Care* 2008;31:2013–2017

16. Boyanov MA, Boneva Z, Christov VG. Testosterone supplementation in men with type 2 diabetes, visceral obesity and partial androgen deficiency. *Aging Male* 2003;6:1–7

17. Kapoor D, Goodwin E, Channer KS, Jones TH. Testosterone replacement therapy improves insulin resistance, glycaemic control, visceral adiposity and hypercholesterolaemia in hypogonadal men with type 2 diabetes. *Eur J Endocrinol* 2006;154:899–906

18. Heufelder AE, Saad F, Bunck MC, Gooren LJ. 52-week treatment with diet and exercise plus transdermal testosterone reverses the metabolic syndrome and improves glycaemic control in men with newly diagnosed type 2 diabetes and subnormal plasma testosterone. *J Androl* 2009;30:726–733

19. Dhindsa S, Ghanim H, Batra M, et al. Insulin resistance and inflammation in hypogonadotropic hypogonadism and their reduction after testosterone replacement in men with type 2 diabetes. *Diabetes Care* 2016;39:1–10

20. Lee CH, Kuo SW, Hung YJ, Hsieh CH, He CT, Yang TC, et al. The effect of testosterone supplement on insulin sensitivity, glucose effectiveness, and acute insulin response after glucose load in male type 2 diabetics. *Endocr Res* 2005;31:139–148

21. Corrales JJ, Almeida M, Burgo R, Mories MT, Miralles JM, Orfao A. Androgen-replacement therapy depresses the ex vivo production of inflammatory cytokines by circulating antigen-presenting cells in aging type-2 diabetic men with partial androgen deficiency. *J Endocrinol* 2006;189:595–604

22. Saad F. The role of testosterone in type 2 diabetes and metabolic syndrome in men. *Arq Bras Endocrinol Metabol* 2009;53:901–907

23. Ding EL, Song Y, Manson JE, et al. Sex hormone-binding globulin and risk of type 2 diabetes in women and men. *N Engl J Med* 2009;361:1152–1163

24. Selvin E, Feinleib M, Zhang L, et al. Androgens and diabetes in men: results from the Third National Health and Nutrition Examination Survey (NHANES III). *Diabetes Care* 2007;30:234–238

25. Lakshman KM, Bhasin S, Araujo AB. Sex hormone-binding globulin as an independent predictor of incident type 2 diabetes mellitus in men. *J Gerontol A Biol Sci Med Sci* 2010;65:503–509

26. Atlantis E, Lange K, Martin S, et al. Testosterone and modifiable risk factors associated with diabetes in men. *Maturitas* 2011;68:279–285

27. Schipf S, Haring R, Friedrich N, et al. Low total testosterone is associated with increased risk of incident type 2 diabetes mellitus in men: Results from the Study of Health in Pomerania (SHIP). *Aging Male* 2011;14:168–175

28. Goto A, Morita A, Goto M, et al. Associations of sex hormone binding globulin and testosterone with diabetes among men and women (the Saku Diabetes Study): a case control study. *Cardiovasc Diabetol* 2012;11:130

29. Kalish GM, Barrett-Connor E, Laughlin GA, Gulanski BI. Association of endogenous sex hormones and insulin resistance among postmenopausal women: results from the Postmenopausal Estrogen/Progestin Intervention Trial. *J Clin Endocrinol Metab* 2003;88:1646–1652

30. Khaw KT, Barrett-Connor E. Fasting plasma glucose levels and endogenous androgens in nondiabetic postmenopausal women. *Clin Sci* (Lond) 1991;80:199–203

31. Phillips GB. Relationship between serum sex hormones and the glucose-insulin-lipid defect in men with obesity. *Metabolism* 1993;42:116–120

32. Kovac JR, Scovell J, Kim ED, Lipshultz LI. A positive role for anabolic androgenic steroids: preventing metabolic syndrome and type 2 diabetes mellitus. *Fertil Steril* 2014;102(1):e5. doi: 10.1016/j.fertnstert.2014.05.010. Epub 4 Jun 2014

33. Bremner WJ, Vitiello MV, Prinz PN. Loss of circadian rhythmicity in blood testosterone levels with aging in normal men. *J Clin Endocrinol Metab* 1983;56:1278–1281

34. Morley JE, Kaiser FE, Perry HM 3rd, et al. Longitudinal changes in testosterone, luteinizing hormone, and follicle-stimulating hormone in healthy older men. *Metabolism* 1997;46:410–413

35. Harman SM, Metter EJ, Tobin JD, Pearson J, Blackman MR; Longitudinal effects of aging on serum total and free testosterone levels in healthy men. Baltimore Longitudinal Study of Aging. *J Clin Endocrinol Metab* 2001;86:724–731

36. Feldman HA, Longcope C, Derby CA, Johannes CB, Araujo AB, Coviello AD, Bremner WJ, McKinlay JB. Age trends in the level of serum testosterone and other hormones in middle-aged men: longitudinal results from the Massachusetts Male Aging Study. *J Clin Endocrinol Metab* 2002;87:589–598

37. Lapauw B, Goemaere S, Zmierczak H, et al. The decline of serum testosterone levels in community-dwelling men over 70 years of age: descriptive data and predictors of longitudinal changes. *Eur J Endocrinol* 2008;159:459–468

38. Bhasin S, Huang G, Travison TG, Basaria S. Age-related changes in the male reproductive axis. In *Endotext* [Internet]. De Groot LJ, Beck-Peccoz P, Chrousos G, Dungan K, Grossman A, Hershman JM, Koch C, McLachlan R, New M, Rebar R, Singer F, Vinik A, Weickert MO, Eds. South Dartmouth, MA, MDText.com, 2000. 14 February 2014

39. Sartorius G, Spasevska S, Idan A, Turner L, Forbes E, Zamojska A, Allan CA, Ly LP, Conway AJ, McLachlan RI, Handelsman DJ. Serum testosterone, dihydrotestosterone and estradiol concentrations in older men self-reporting very good health: the Healthy Man Study. *Clin Endocrinol* 2012;77:755–763

40. Basaria S, Coviello AD, Travison TG, et al. Adverse events associated with testosterone administration. *N Engl J Med* 2010;363:109–122

41. U.S. Food and Drug Administration, Center for Drug Evaluation and Research. Minutes of the Joint Meeting of the Bone, Reproductive and Urologic Drugs Advisory Committee and the Drug Safety and Risk Man-

agement Advisory Committee, September 17, 2014. Washington, DC, FDA, 2014. Available from http://www.fda.gov/downloads/AdvisoryCommittees/ CommitteesMeetingMaterials/Drugs/ReproductiveHealth DrugsAdvisory-Committee/UCM418144.pdf

42. Crandall J, Schade D, Ma Y, et al. The influence of age on the effects of lifestyle modification and metformin in prevention of diabetes. *J Gerontol A Biol Sci Med Sci* 2006;61:1075–1081

43. Basaria S, Muller DC, Carducci MA, Egan J, Dobs AS. Hyperglycemia and insulin resistance in men with prostate carcinoma who receive androgen-deprivation therapy. *Cancer* 2006;106:581–588

44. Keating NL, O'Malley JO, Smith MR. Diabetes and cardiovascular disease during androgen deprivation therapy for prostate cancer. *J Clin Oncol* 2006;24:4448–4456

45. Smith MR. Androgen deprivation therapy and risk for diabetes and cardiovascular disease in prostate cancer survivors. *Curr Urol Rep* 2008;9:197–202

46. Keating NL, O'Malley AJ, Freedland SJ, Smith MR. Diabetes and cardiovascular disease during androgen deprivation therapy: observational study of veterans with prostate cancer. *J Natl Cancer Inst* 2010;102:39–46

47. Keating NL, Liu PH, O'Malley AJ, Freedland SJ, Smith MR. Androgen-deprivation therapy and diabetes control among diabetic men with prostate cancer. *Eur Urol* 2014;65:816–824

48. Levine GN, D'Amico AV, Berger P, Clark PE, Eckel RH, Keating NL, Milani RV, Sagalowsky AI, Smith MR, Zakai N; American Heart Association Council on Clinical Cardiology and Council on Epidemiology and Prevention, the American Cancer Society, and the American Urological Association. Androgen-deprivation therapy in prostate cancer and cardiovascular risk: a science advisory from the American Heart Association, American Cancer Society, and American Urological Association: endorsed by the American Society for Radiation Oncology. *CA Cancer J Clin* 2010;60:194–201

49. U.S. Food and Drug Administration. Drug safety communication 10-20-2010: Update to ongoing safety review of GnRH agonists and notification to manufacturers of GnRH agonists to add new safety information to labeling regarding increased risk of diabetes and certain cardiovascular diseases, 2010. Available from http://www.fda.gov/Drugs/DrugSafety/ucm229986.htm

50. Smith JC, Bennett S, Evans LM, et al. The effects of induced hypogonadism on arterial stiffness, body composition, and metabolic parameters in males with prostate cancer. *J Clin Endocrinol Metab* 2001;86:4261–4267

51. Berruti A, Dogliotti L, Terrone C, et al. Gruppo Onco Urologico Piemontese (G.O.U.P.), Rete Oncologica Piemontese. Changes in bone mineral density, lean body mass and fat content as measured by dual energy x-ray absorptiometry in patients with prostate cancer without apparent bone metastases given androgen deprivation therapy. *J Urol* 2002;167:2361–2367

52. Lee H, McGovern K, Finkelstein JS, Smith MR. Changes in bone mineral density and body composition during initial and long-term gonadotropin releasing hormone agonist treatment for prostate carcinoma. *Cancer* 2005;104:1633–1637

53. Smith MR, Lee H, McGovern F, et al. Metabolic changes during gonadotropin-releasing hormone agonist therapy for prostate cancer: differences from the classic metabolic syndrome. *Cancer* 2008;112:2188–2194

54. Smith MR, Lee H, Nathan DM. Insulin sensitivity during combined androgen blockade for prostate cancer. *J Clin Endocrinol Metab* 2006;91:1305–1308

55. Eri LM, Urdal P, Bechensteen AG. Effects of the luteinizing hormone-releasing hormone agonist leuprolide on lipoproteins, fibrinogen and plasminogen activator inhibitor in patients with benign prostatic hyperplasia. *J Urol* 1995;154:100–104

5

Antihypertensive Agents

Most antihypertensive medications in current use are generally well tolerated, such that no particular class of agents is specifically contraindicated in patients with diabetes. Diuretics and β-blockers have been well documented to reduce cardiovascular morbidity and mortality in the general hypertensive population.[1] Moreover, secondary prevention studies have confirmed the efficacy of β-blockers in preventing reinfarction and sudden death in patients with a previous history of myocardial infarction,[2] as well as the survival advantage of angiotensin-converting enzyme (ACE) inhibitors in patients with heart failure.[3]

DIURETICS

Several studies have shown that thiazide diuretics induce insulin resistance in hypertensive patients,[4,5] and may be associated with treatment-emergent diabetes.[6] In both the Systolic Hypertension in the Elderly Patients (SHEP) and the Antihypertensive and Lipid-Lowering Treatment to Prevent Heart Attack Trial (ALLHAT) trials, treatment with chlorthalidone was associated with increased rates of incident diabetes compared to placebo (SHEP) or other active agents (ALLHAT) during a 3- to 4-year follow-up period.[7] The magnitude of diabetes risk was ~18% to 49% for chlorthalidone versus comparators. In the Anglo-Scandinavian Cardiac Outcomes Trial (ASCOT), the rate of incident diabetes was ~30% higher in the thiazide-containing treatment arm compared with the calcium-channel blocker (CCB)–ACE inhibitor arm.[8] Diuretics also have been associated with unfavorable changes in serum lipoprotein fractions, principally elevated triglycerides and decreased high-density lipoprotein (HDL) cholesterol levels, which appear to be transient. Insulin resistance and impaired insulin secretion, probably mediated by hypokalemia, appear to underlie the mechanism of the dysglycemia associated with thiazide and thiazide-like diuretics.[9,10] Other proposed mechanisms include increased free fatty acids and increased hepatic glucose output.[11,12] As the metabolic effects of thiazide diuretics may be dose related, use of smaller doses (e.g., 6.25–25 mg) is advisable.

DOI: 10.2337/9781580406192.05   **47**

β-ADRENORECEPTOR BLOCKERS

Both selective and nonselective β-blockers can induce insulin resistance[4,5] and increase diabetes risk. In the Atherosclerosis Risk in Communities (ARIC) study, the rate of incident diabetes was 28% higher in hypertensive patients treated with β-blockers compared with an untreated control group.[13] Reports from other recent trials also document the increased risk of diabetes associated with the use of β-blockers (reviewed by McCullen and Ahmed[14]). During hyperinsulinemic euglycemic clamp studies, patients without diabetes treated with metoprolol (200 mg/day) or atenolol (50–100 mg/day) for 4–6 months had ~25% reduction in insulin sensitivity.[5] Evidence also indicates that β-blockers can alter insulin clearance,[15] reduce insulin secretion,[16] promote weight gain,[17] and decrease peripheral blood flow,[14] all of which are mechanisms that could increase diabetes risk. These reports, however, have not been widely replicated, and the glycemic effects of the reported alterations in insulin sensitivity and secretion are either modest or unapparent in the majority of patients treated with β-blockers. Thus, the exact mechanisms for induction of diabetes by β-blockers remain to be elucidated.

Parenthetically, in diabetic patients, β-blockers can mask hypoglycemic symptoms[18] and prolong recovery from insulin-induced hypoglycemia. Furthermore, β-blockers have been associated with unfavorable changes in serum lipoprotein fractions, including elevated triglycerides and decreased HDL cholesterol levels. Drugs with combined β- and α-adrenergic blocking activity (e.g., labetalol, carvedilol) might have a less adverse metabolic profile compared with pure β-blockers.[19]

α-ADRENORECEPTOR BLOCKERS

α_1-Blockers, such as prazosin and terazosin, and combined α- and β-blockers (labetalol and carvedilol) have been reported consistently to decrease insulin resistance and improve glucose tolerance.[1,2]

ANGIOTENSIN-CONVERTING ENZYME INHIBITORS AND ANGIOTENSIN RECEPTOR BLOCKERS

Overactivity of the renin-angiotensin-aldosterone system has been associated with cellular and molecular changes that lead to insulin resistance and impaired β-cell function.[20,21] Moreover, evidence shows that ACE inhibitors can improve insulin sensitivity.[5,22] Consonant with these reports, post hoc analyses from several multicenter randomized controlled studies have observed significant reductions in the incidence of type 2 diabetes (T2D) in hypertensive patients treated with either ACE inhibitors or angiotensin receptor blockers (ARBs) compared with other agents, such as thiazide diuretics or β-blockers.[8,21,23,24] A randomized trial of the protective effects of ramipril (vs. placebo) on diabetes showed an increased rate of reversion from prediabetes to normoglycemia but not a reduction in new-onset diabetes among subjects with prediabetes in the ramipril arm.[25] In the NAVIGATOR trial, however, subjects with prediabetes randomized to valsartan treatment showed a 14% decrease in the incidence of T2D compared with placebo.[26]

A network meta-analysis (Figure 5.1) of 22 clinical trials, that enrolled a total of 143,153 participants who did not have diabetes at randomization, suggests a hierarchy of diabetes risk from different antihypertensive agents. In that report, the association of antihypertensive drugs with incident diabetes was lowest for ARB and ACE inhibitors followed by CCBs, placebo, β-blockers, and diuretics, in that order.[27]

Thus, it is certain that ACE inhibitors and ARBs do not increase diabetes risk, and it is quite probable that they decrease risk. ACE inhibitors and ARBs are generally well tolerated by diabetic patients and are specifically indicated for nephroprotection in patients with microalbuminuria. These agents also confer significant cardiovascular benefits. Note, however, that angiotensin inhibition may precipitate acute renal failure in patients with bilateral atherosclerotic renovascular disease or may exacerbate hyperkalemia in patients with diabetes-associated type IV renal tubular acidosis. Furthermore, these agents should be used with caution in patients with diabetic autonomic neuropathy, who may respond with a worsening of orthostatic symptoms.

CALCIUM CHANNEL BLOCKERS

There have been anecdotal reports of hyperglycemia[28] or improved glucose tolerance[29] in some patients treated with the verapamil. In general, however, clinical use of CCBs does not pose a significant diabetes risk and is associated with neutral effects on glucose tolerance and insulin sensitivity.[5,22,27]

DIAZOXIDE AND OTHER PERIPHERAL VASODILATORS

The potent arteriolar vasodilator diazoxide causes hyperglycemia principally by inhibiting insulin secretion.[30] Other suggested mechanisms for induction of hyper-

Figure 5.1—Meta-analysis of incident diabetes in antihypertensive drug trials. *Source:* Modified from Elliott and Meyer.[27]

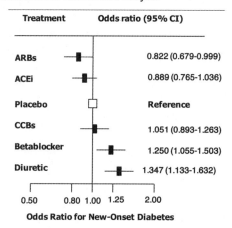

Treatment	Odds ratio (95% CI)
ARBs	0.822 (0.679-0.999)
ACEi	0.889 (0.765-1.036)
Placebo	Reference
CCBs	1.051 (0.893-1.263)
Betablocker	1.250 (1.055-1.503)
Diuretic	1.347 (1.133-1.632)

0.50   0.80 1.00 1.25   2.00

Odds Ratio for New-Onset Diabetes

glycemia include activation of sympathetic discharge and increased gluconeogenesis. Diazoxide is indicated as an adjunctive treatment for insulinoma and also has been used to reverse pentamidine-induced hypoglycemia. Diazoxide inhibits insulin secretion by opening the K_{ATP} channels on the β-cell membrane, which maintains hyperpolarization and prevents calcium entry into the cell. Although the acute effect of diazoxide inhibition of insulin secretion is hyperglycemia, over time, diazoxide inhibits pancreatic β-cell apoptosis and actually decreases diabetes risk.[31-33] The acute effect of diazoxide has been exploited therapeutically for the reversal of pentamidine-induced hypoglycemia.[34]

Minoxidil has been associated with exacerbation of glucose intolerance in patients with diabetes and in people with impaired glucose tolerance.[35] Like diazoxide, the vasodilatory effect of minoxidil provokes an adrenergic response that potentially could lead to catecholamine-induced hyperglycemia. No such dysglycemic effect has been reported for hydralazine, which in fact has neutral or favorable effects on plasma lipoprotein profiles.[1,36,37]

OTHER AGENTS

The centrally acting antihypertensive agents guanabenz, guanfacine, and clonidine are not associated with adverse effects on carbohydrate or lipid metabolism.

REFERENCES

1. Alderman MH. Which antihypertensive agent first—and why! *JAMA* 1992;267:2786–2787

2. Yusuf S, Wittes J, Probstfield J. Evaluating effects of treatment in subgroups of patients within a clinical trial: the case of non-Q-wave myocardial infarction and β-blockers. *Am J Cardiol* 1990;66:220–222

3. SOLVD Investigators. Effect of enalapril on survival in patients with reduced left ventricular ejection fractions and congestive heart failure. *N Engl J Med* 1991;325:293–302

4. Pollare T, Lithell H, Berne C. A comparison of the effects of hydrochlorothiazide and captopril on glucose and lipid metabolism in patients with hypertension. *N Engl J Med* 1989;321:868–873

5. Lithell HOL. Effect of antihypertensive drugs on insulin, glucose, and lipid metabolism. *Diabetes Care* 1991;14:203–209

6. Sowers JR. Hypertension in type 2 diabetes: update on therapy. *J Clin Hypertens* 1994;1:41–47

7. Sierra C, Ruilope LM. New-onset diabetes and antihypertensive therapy: comments on ALLHAT trial. *J Renin-Angiotensin-Aldosterone Syst* 2003;4:169–170

8. Dahlof B, Sever PS, Poulter NR, et al. Prevention of cardiovascular events with an antihypertensive regimen of amlodipine adding perindopril as required versus atenolol adding bendroflumethiazide as required, in the Anglo-Scandinavian Cardiac Outcomes Trial–Blood Pressure Lowering Arm (ASCOT-BPLA): a multicentre randomised controlled trial. *Lancet* 2005;366:895–906

9. Gulliford MC, Charlton J, Latinovic R. Trends in antihypertensive and lipid lowering therapy in subjects with type II diabetes: clinical effectiveness or clinical discretion? *J Human Hypertens* 2005;19:111–117

10. Zillich AJ, Garg J, Basu S, Bakris GL, Carter BL. Thiazide diuretics, potassium, and the development of diabetes: a quantitative review. *Hypertension* 2006;48:219–224

11. Flamenbaum W. Metabolic consequences of antihypertensive therapy. *Ann Intern Med* 1983;98:875–880

12. Weir MR, Moser M. Diuretics and β-blockers: is there a risk for dyslipidemia? *Am Heart J* 2000;139:174–183

13. Gress TW, Nieto FJ, Shahar E, Wofford MR, Brancati FL. Hypertension and antihypertensive therapy as risk factors for type 2 diabetes mellitus. *N Engl J Med* 2000;342:905–912

14. McCullen MK, Ahmed I. Drug-induced hyperglycemia and diabetes mellitus. In *Type 2 Diabetes, Principles and Practice*. 2nd ed. Goldstein BJ and Müller-Wieland D, Eds. Taylor & Francis, New York, 2007, p. 513–528

15. Chan JC, Cockram CS, Critchley JA. Drug-induced disorders of glucose metabolism: mechanisms and management. *Drug Safety* 1996;15:135–157

16. Van Bortel LM, Ament AJ. Selective versus nonselective β-adrenoceptor antagonists in hypertension. *Pharmacoeconomics* 1995;8:513–523

17. Pischon T, Sharma AM. Use of β-blockers in obesity, hypertension: potential role of weight gain. *Obes Rev* 2001;2:275–280

18. Hirsch IB, Boyle PJ, Craft S, Cryer PE. Higher glycemic thresholds for symptoms during β-adrenergic blockade in IDDM. *Diabetes* 1991;40:1177–1186

19. Bakris GL, Fonseca V, Katholi RE, et al. Metabolic effects of carvedilol vs. metoprolol in patients with type 2 diabetes mellitus and hypertension: a randomized controlled trial. *JAMA* 2004;292:2227–2236

20. Ferrannini E, Gastaldelli A, Miyazaki Y, Matsuda M, Pettiti M, Natali A, Mari A, DeFronzo RA. Predominant role of reduced β-cell sensitivity to glucose over insulin resistance in impaired glucose tolerance. *Diabetologia* 2003;46:1211–1219

21. Jandeleit-Dahm KA, Tikellis C, Reid CM, Johnston CI, Cooper ME. Why blockade of the renin-angiotensin system reduces the incidence of new-onset diabetes. *J Hypertens* 2005;23:463–473

22. Giordano M, Matsuda M, Sanders L, Canessa ML, DeFronzo RA. Effects of angiotensin-converting enzyme inhibitors, Ca^{2+} channel antagonists, and a-adrenergic blockers on glucose and lipid metabolism in NIDDM patients with hypertension. *Diabetes* 1995;44:665–671

23. Yusuf S, Sleight P, Pogue J, Bosch J, Davies R, Dagenais G. Effects of an angiotensin-converting-enzyme inhibitor, ramipril, on cardiovascular events in high-risk patients. The Heart Outcomes Prevention Evaluation Study Investigators. *N Engl J Med* 2000;342:145–153

24. Barzilay JI, Davis BR, Cutler JA, et al. Fasting glucose levels and incident diabetes mellitus in older nondiabetic adults randomized to receive 3 different classes of antihypertensive treatment: a report from the Antihypertensive and Lipid-Lowering Treatment to Prevent Heart Attack Trial (ALLHAT). *Arch Intern Med* 2006;166:2191–2201

25. Bosch J, Yusuf S, Gerstein HC, et al. Effect of ramipril on the incidence of diabetes. *N Engl J Med* 2006;355:1551–1562

26. NAVIGATOR Study Group. Effect of valsartan on the incidence of diabetes and cardiovascular events [published correction appears in *N Engl J Med* 2010;362:1748]. *N Engl J Med* 2010;362:1477–1490

27. Elliott WJ, Meyer PM. Incident diabetes in clinical trials of antihypertensive drugs: a network meta-analysis. *Lancet* 2007;369:201–207

28. Roth AM, Belhassen B, Laniado S. Slow-release verapamil and hyperglycemic metabolic acidosis. *Ann Intern Med* 1989;110:171–172

29. Andersson DE, Rojdmark S. Improvement of glucose tolerance by verapamil in patients with non-insulin-dependent diabetes mellitus. *Acta Med Scand* 1981;210:27–33

30. Zunkler BL, Lenzen S, Manner K, Panten U, Trube G. Concentration-dependent effects of tolbutamide, meglitinide, glipizide, glibenclamide and diazoxide on ATP-regulated K^+ currents in pancreatic B-cells. *Naunyn Schmiedebergs Arch Pharmacol* 1988;337:225–230

31. Guldstrand M, Grill V, Bjorklund A, Lins PE, Adamson U. Improved B-cell function after short-term treatment with diazoxide in obese subjects with type 2 diabetes. *Diabetes Metab* 2002;28:448–456

32. Hansen JB, Arkhammer PO, Bodvarsdottir TB, Wahl P. Inhibition of insulin secretion as a new drug target in the treatment of metabolic disorders. *Curr Med Chem* 2004;11:1595–1615

33. Huang Q, Bu S, Yu Y, Guo Z, et al. Diazoxide prevents diabetes through inhibiting pancreatic B-cells from apoptosis via Bcl-2/Bax rate and p38-B mitogen-activated protein kinase. *Endocrinology* 2007;148:81–91

34. Fitzgerald DB, Young IS. Reversal of pentamidine-induced hypoglycaemia with oral diazoxide. *J Trop Med Hyg* 1984;87:15–19

35. Lederballe Pedersen O. Long-term experience with minoxidil in combination treatment of severe arterial hypertension. *Acta Cardiol* 1977;32:283–293

36. Ames RP. The effects of antihypertensive drugs on serum lipids and lipoproteins II. Non-diuretic drugs. *Drugs* 1986;32:335–357

37. Wandell PE, Brorsson B, Aberg H. Drug use in patients with diabetes. *Diabetes Care* 1996;19:992–994

6

Catecholamines, β-Adrenergic Agonists, and Bronchodilators

S ome of the drugs used for the treatment of asthma and chronic obstructive pulmonary disease, such as β-adrenergic agonists and methylxanthines, can have appreciable effects on carbohydrate metabolism.

β-ADRENERGIC AGONISTS

Catecholamines and $β_2$-adrenergic agonists stimulate glycogenolysis and lipolysis, and transiently increase insulin and glucagon secretion.[1-3] These agents also induce insulin resistance and decrease peripheral glucose utilization.[4] The net effect of these actions is elevated plasma concentrations of glucose, lactate, and nonesterified fatty acids (NEFAs). The catecholamine-induced insulin resistance is mediated, in part, by increased NEFAs from lipolysis and by direct interference with the insulin receptor and postreceptor signaling mechanisms.[5] Epinephrine, isoproterenol, terbutaline, and over-the-counter decongestants containing sympathomimetic drugs are capable of elevating blood glucose. Inhaled agents are far less likely to affect glucose metabolism compared with oral or parenteral medications.

THEOPHYLLINE

Therapeutic concentrations of theophylline can increase plasma catecholamine levels and thereby lead to increased lipolysis and release of NEFAs.[6] Thus, theophylline can induce hyperglycemia through the well-known diabetogenic effects of catecholamines and increased NEFAs. Theophylline-induced hypokalemia also could be a contributory factor, especially in cases of overdose.[7] These actions of theophylline and other xanthines may be mediated by inhibition of phosphodiesterase, leading to potentiation of catecholamine action.[8] Very high doses of theophylline stimulate insulin secretion probably by an indirect β-adrenergic mechanism, but this is not seen with standard doses.[6]

REFERENCES

1. Mayer S, Moran NC, Fain J. The effects of adrenergic blocking agents on some metabolic actions of catecholamines. *J Pharmacol Exp Therapeutics* 1961;134:18–27

2. Young JB, Langsberg L. Adrenergic influence on peripheral hormone secretion. In *Adrenoceptors and Catecholamine Action. Part B.* Kunos G, Ed. New York, John Wiley & Sons, 1983, p. 157–217

3. Halter JB, Beard JC, Porte D Jr. Islet function and stress hyperglycemia: plasma glucose and epinephrine interaction. *Am J Physiol Endocrinol Metab* 1984;247:E47–E52

4. Rizza RA, Cryer PE, Haymond MW, Gerich JE. Adrenergic mechanisms of catecholamine action on glucose homeostasis in man. *Metabolism* 1980; 29(11 Suppl. 1):1155–1163

5. Kirsch DM, Baumgarten M, Deufel T, Rinninger F, Kemmler W, Häring HU. Catecholamine-induced insulin resistance of glucose transport in isolated rat adipocytes. *Biochem J* 1983;216:737–745

6. Vestal RE, Eriksson CE, Musser B, Ozaki LK, Halter JB. Effect of intravenous aminophylline on plasma levels of catecholamines and related cardiovascular and metabolic responses in man. *Circulation* 1983;67:162–171

7. Chan JC, Cockram CS. Drug-induced disturbances of carbohydrate metabolism. *Adverse Drug React Toxicol Rev* 1991;10:1–29

8. Hall KW, Dobson KE, Dalton JG, Ghignone MC, Penner SB. Metabolic abnormalities associated with intentional theophylline overdose. *Ann Intern Med* 1984;101:457–462

7

Lipid-Lowering Drugs

With regard to blood glucose regulation, the collective evidence indicates that fibrates and bile acid sequestrants may have beneficial effects, statins have a variable effect, and nicotinic acid increases the risk for dysglycemia. Furthermore, emerging data suggest that, in addition to their well-known cardioprotective effects, statins and fibrates might decrease the risk for diabetic microvascular complications (e.g., retinopathy, nephropathy, neuropathy).

NICOTINIC ACID

Some patients with dyslipidemia receiving chronic treatment with nicotinic acid experience a worsening of glucose tolerance.[1] People with prediabetes or diabetes appear to be at greater risk of glycemic exacerbation following exposure to nicotinic acid.[2] Despite many decades of clinical use for the treatment of dyslipidemia, the mechanism of action of nicotinic acid is not fully understood. The discovery of GPR109A (a Gi-protein-coupled receptor expressed predominantly in fat cells) as a high-affinity receptor for nicotinic acid[3,4] is an important step toward greater understanding of the cellular actions of nicotinic acid.[5,6] Activation of GPR109A through agonist binding by nicotinic acid leads to the inhibition of hormone-sensitive lipase, which results in decreased lipolysis and a fall in circulating nonesterified fatty acids (NEFA) levels. [3-6] The downstream pathways linking decreased NEFA to the typical lipid effects of nicotinic acid (namely, decreases in triglycerides and low-density lipoprotein [LDL] cholesterol and increased high-density lipoprotein [HDL] cholesterol levels), though unclear, could involve inhibition of de novo hepatic lipogenesis via inhibition of diacylglycerol-acetyl transferase 2.[7,8]

Nicotinic acid has complex interactions with glucoregulatory physiology. Acutely, it inhibits lipolysis, decreases NEFA levels, and improves insulin sensitivity by stimulating peripheral glucose uptake and oxidation.[9] Long-term treatment with nicotinic acid, however, results in rebound lipolysis, increased NEFA levels, insulin resistance, increased gluconeogenesis, with resultant dysglycemia.[2,10-14] These adverse metabolic effects of nicotinic acid are dose-dependent,[15] and the clinical impact on glycemic control in patients receiving antidiabetic medications appears to be modest (~0.2 % increase in HbA_{1c}).[16] Sustained-release formulation of nicotinic acid has been reported to be associated with less perturbation of glucose tolerance, but the risk is not negligible.[17-19]

DOI: 10.2337/9781580406192.07

In the Heart Protection Study 2–Treatment of HDL to Reduce the Incidence of Vascular Events (HPS2-THRIVE) study,[19] 25,673 adults with vascular disease were randomly assigned to receive 2 g of extended-release niacin and 40 mg of laropiprant or a matching placebo daily. During a follow-up period of ~4 years, among the 17,374 participants who did not have diabetes at baseline, treatment with niacin–laropiprant, as compared with placebo, was associated with a 32% proportional increase in new diabetes diagnoses, although the absolute rates were low (5.7% vs. 4.3%, $P < 0.001$). Furthermore, treatment with niacin–laropiprant was associated with a significant risk of deterioration of glycemic control among the 8,299 participants who had diabetes at baseline.

Approach to Management and Risk Reduction

Nicotinic acid is strictly not contraindicated in patients with diabetes, but physicians should be attentive to the risk of treatment-emergent worsening of glycemic control. Nicotinic acid has a beneficial profile in its ability to raise plasma HDL cholesterol levels and decrease the levels of total cholesterol. Unlike the statin drugs, however, the lipid effects of nicotinic acid did not translate to a reduction in major vascular events (nonfatal myocardial infarction, death from coronary causes, stroke, or arterial revascularization), as compared with placebo, in the HPS2-THRIVE study.[19] Thus, the rationale for prescribing nicotinic acid instead of a statin drug in the management of dyslipidemia needs to be well justified and compelling.

If nicotinic acid is used to treat dyslipidemia in diabetic patients, careful monitoring and optimization of glycemic control is advisable. Because of the dose-related dysglycemic effect,[15] use of lower doses (~1,000–1,500 mg/day) of nicotinic acid is recommended in people with diabetes.[18] In people without a history of diabetes, it is prudent to obtain plasma glucose levels before initiation of nicotinic acid therapy, to identify people with prediabetes. Because people with prediabetes have an increased risk for hyperglycemia following exposure to nicotinic acid,[2] they should receive diabetes prevention counseling and preferably should be treated with submaximal doses of nicotinic acid as a second-line option, if other agents for control of dyslipidemia are not tolerated.

STATINS

In addition to the well-known cholesterol-lowering effects, statin therapy has been associated with beneficial *pleiotropic* effects, including reduction of circulating inflammatory and oxidative stress markers, and improvement of endothelial function. The expectations that these effects would have a favorable impact on diabetes risk have not been borne out by clinical trials. Instead, some studies have reported an increased risk of diabetes in statin-treated patients, although the data are conflicting.

In the JUPITER trial that demonstrated superior efficacy of rosuvastatin over placebo in decreasing cardiovascular events among subjects with elevated C-reactive protein, the rosuvastatin group had a higher incidence of physician-reported diabetes than placebo (3.0% vs. 2.4% during a median follow-up period of 1.9 years).[20] A similar trend has been reported for other statins.[21] In the Women's Health Initiative (WHI), which recruited 161,808 postmenopausal women ages 50–79 years old between 1993 and 1998, analysis of data collected through 2005, including nearly 153,840 women without diabetes at enrollment, found that 7.04% (~11,000) reported taking statins.[22] A total of 10,242 incident cases of self-reported diabetes occurred during 1,004,466 person-years of follow-up. Among statin-treated women, 9.9% self-reported diabetes diagnosis, compared with 6.4% of women who did not report taking statins.[22] The authors calculated that statin use was associated with an increased relative risk of diabetes (hazard ratio [HR] 1.71 [95% confidence interval, CI, 1.61–1.83]). The association was observed for all types of statin medications and remained significant after adjusting for potential confounders (multivariate-adjusted HR 1.48 [95% CI 1.38–1.59]).

In the Metabolic Syndrome in Men (METSIM) cohort study, which followed 8,749 men (ages 45–73 years old) who initially did not have diabetes for 5.9 years, 625 new cases of diabetes were diagnosed. Of the cohort, 2,142 men were receiving treatment with statins and 6,607 men had no history of statin use. The authors report a hazard ratio for diabetes of 1.46 (95% CI 1.22–1.74) for people using statins compared with nonusers.[23]

In contrast to the findings in the aforementioned JUPITER, WHI, and METSIM cohort studies, a meta-analysis that included 42,860 patients without preexisting diabetes, who were randomized to statins versus placebo and follow-up for 4 years, reported no increased hazard of statin-induced diabetes.[24] Similarly, a nested case–control analysis of the U.K.-based General Practice Research Database found no increased risk of diabetes associated with statin use.[25] In yet another meta-analysis, there was a reported 9% increased risk for new onset diabetes associated with statin therapy; older participants had a higher risk of diabetes with statin use ($P = 0.019$), but, surprisingly, adiposity (baseline BMI) was not a predictor of the increased diabetes risk.[26]

The mechanisms of the reported statin-associated increase in diabetes risk are not well known. Potential or suggested mechanisms include HMG-coenzyme A reductase inhibition leading to weight gain and insulin resistance,[23,27] decreased expression of glucose transporter (GLUT4),[28] and impaired insulin secretion,[23,29] among others.[30] These suggested mechanisms, largely deduced from in vitro preclinical experiments, do not fully explain the heterogeneity and peculiarities of the diabetes risk associated with statin exposure in humans. Clearly, further studies are needed to elucidate the exact mechanisms, and potentially to delineate specific risk factors, for statin-associated risk of dysglycemia. Among patients with established diabetes, statin treatment is associated with modest to minimal change in HbA_{1c} levels, based on a random-effects model meta-analysis of pooled data from nine trials involving 9,696 participants (4,980 statin, 4,716 control) followed for 3.6 years.[31] In that analysis, the mean HbA_{1c} of participants randomized to statins was 0.12% (1.3 mmol/mol) higher than those randomized to the control group.[31] In 2012, the U.S. Food and Drug Administration (FDA) added new safety label changes for the statin class of cholesterol-lowering drugs regarding the potential for increased hemoglobin A_{1c} and fasting plasma glucose levels.[32]

Approach to Risk Reduction

The available published data on the association between statin use and increased diabetes risk are somewhat inconsistent. The most informative of the available data sources on the subject seems to be the prospective, randomized, controlled JUPITER trial.[20] Unlike other studies, diabetes was a prespecified outcome measure and was based on physician diagnosis (rather than self-report) in the JUPITER trial. The JUPITER study found an absolute difference of 0.6% in the risk of incident physician-diagnosed diabetes in patients assigned to rosuvastatin compared with placebo (3.0% vs. 2.4%). That finding from the JUPITER study together with the absolute difference of 3.6% increase in self-reported diabetes among women who reported using statin drugs in the WHI[22] would suggest that statin-associated diabetes is an infrequent clinical event. Among people with preexisting diabetes, given the minimal alterations that occur in plasma glucose levels following statin exposure,[31] no special treatment is warranted besides adherence to recommended standards of care.[33]

In a risk–benefit analysis of the JUPITER cohort,[34] participants were stratified on the basis of four major risk factors for developing diabetes: metabolic syndrome, impaired fasting glucose, BMI ≥ 30 kg/m^2, or HbA$_{1c}$ ≥ 6%. Strikingly, the participants with one or more major diabetes risk factor had a 10.5-fold greater risk of developing diabetes during up to 5 years of follow-up (incidence rate 1.88 vs. 0.18 per 100 person-years; HR 10.5 [95% CI 6.98–15.8]; $P = 0.001$).[34] Compared with placebo, the average time to diagnosis of diabetes was accelerated by 5.4 weeks in the statin group (84.3 $\pm$ 47.8 weeks on rosuvastatin vs. 89.7 $\pm$ 50.4 weeks on placebo) and statin treatment was associated with a 25% increase in diabetes (270 reports of diabetes vs. 216 in the placebo group; HR 1.25 [95% CI 1.05–1.49]; $P = 0.01$) during ~5 years of follow-up.[34] To place this in perspective, participants assigned to the placebo arm of the Diabetes Prevention Program (who harbored risk factors, such as impaired glucose tolerance, high-normal fasting plasma glucose, overweight/obesity, and metabolic syndrome), had ~30% cumulative incidence of type 2 diabetes (T2D) during ~3 years of follow-up.[35]

Although current knowledge of the susceptibility risk factors for statin-associated diabetes is incomplete, the data from JUPITER and other reports support the use of the standard diabetes risk factors (Table 1.1) when counseling candidates for statin therapy who do not have diabetes.[23,27,28,34] Thus, careful documentation of diabetes risk factors and blood glucose screening for diabetes seem appropriate before the initiation of statin therapy. Such an approach would identify people with undiagnosed diabetes and high-risk individuals, including those with prediabetes. Because emerging information suggests that weight gain and insulin resistance might be mechanisms linking statin use and dysglycemia,[23,27,28] lifestyle counseling for diabetes prevention (see Chapter 12) is recommended as a general practice when prescribing statins for people with prediabetes, people who are overweight, and those who meet criteria for the metabolic syndrome.

Regarding cardiovascular benefits, the JUPITER participants with one or more diabetes risk factors, who were allocated to rosuvastatin treatment, experienced a 39% reduction in the primary endpoint (myocardial infarction, stroke, admission to hospital for unstable angina, arterial revascularization, or cardiovascular death), a 36% reduction in venous thromboembolism, a 17% reduction in total mortality, and a 28% increase in diabetes.[34] For participants with no major diabetes risk factor, allocation to statin treatment was associated with a 52% reduction in the primary endpoint, a 53% reduction in venous thromboembolism, a 22% reduction in total mortality, and no increase in diabetes. Thus, the presence of preexisting diabetes risk factors (such as obesity, prediabetes, and metabolic syndrome) was predictive of statin treatment–emergent diabetes in the JUPITER trial.

Notably, the JUPITER participants who developed diabetes during follow-up ($n = 270$ on rosuvastatin; $n = 216$ on placebo) had cardiovascular risk reduction from statin therapy that was comparable to that seen in the trial as a whole. Among participants with no diabetes risk factors, a total of 86 vascular events or deaths were avoided with no new cases of diabetes diagnosed; among those with one or more risk factors, the authors calculated that 134 vascular events or deaths were avoided for every 54 new cases of diabetes diagnosed.[34] Sattar et al.[26] in their meta-analysis calculated that 255 patients treated with statins for 4 years would result in 1 case of diabetes but 5.4 fewer coronary events. On the basis of such a favorable profile, the benefits of statins clearly outweigh the small potential risk of incident diabetes.

FIBRATES

Hypertriglyceridemia is a hallmark of diabetic dyslipidemia, and fibrates (gem-fibrozil, fenofibrate, bezafibrate) are frequently prescribed to control it. A retrospective analysis of a large database showed that exposure to bezafibrate was specifically associated with reduced risk of incident diabetes.[36] The database was composed of 12,161 patients who were treated with bezafibrate and 4,191 patients treated with other fibrates; baseline characteristics were similar between the two groups. The hazard ratio for incident diabetes was 0.66 (95% CI 0.53–0.81) among bezafibrate users compared with users of other fibrates. The protective effect of bezafibrate became stronger with increasing duration of therapy. The potential mechanisms for prevention of diabetes might be amelioration of insulin resistance[37] through dual activation of peroxisome proliferator–activated receptor α- and γ-receptors.[38] Clearly, randomized controlled trials are needed before bezafibrate or other fibrates can be recommended specifically for the prevention of diabetes.

COLESEVELAM AND BILE ACID SEQUESTRANTS

The bile acid sequestrant colesevelam is the only cholesterol-lowering agent that has been approved by the FDA for the adjunctive treatment of T2D. In a randomized, placebo-controlled study in patients with T2D who were poorly controlled with metformin, the addition of colesevelam (3.75 g/day) reduced HbA$_{1c}$ by 0.54% compared with placebo during a 26-week follow-up period.[39] The mechanisms whereby colesevelam improves glycemic control are unclear. Bile acid sequestrants are not absorbed systemically, but they exert their lipid-lowering effects by binding bile acids in the gut. The resultant exclusion of bile acids from the enterohepatic circulation leads to increased hepatic bile acid synthesis. The latter process is catalyzed by cholesterol 7-α-hydroxylase, which utilizes cholesterol as substrate, resulting in a depletion of the LDL cholesterol pool. Recent advances in our understanding of bile acids indicate that these moieties exert diverse metabolic effects through tightly regulated signaling pathways.[40] It is plausible that interference with bile acid signal transduction plays a role in the effects of colesevelam and other bile acid sequestrants on glucose metabolism.[40]

LIPID-LOWERING DRUGS AND DIABETES COMPLICATIONS

The protective effects of statins and, to some extent, fibrates on cardiovascular disease have been well documented. Emerging data also suggest that the use of statins and fibrates may be associated with a decreased risk for diabetic microvascular complications. In an observational study, Davis et al.[41] reported that the risk of developing peripheral neuropathy among patients with diabetes who were treated with statins was decreased by 35%, and decreased by 48% in those taking fibrates, compared with patients not treated with statins or fibrates. The benefits seen with statins and fibrates on diabetic neuropathy appeared specific to each drug class and were independent of their effects on plasma lipid profiles. In the Fenofibrate and Event Lowering in Diabetes (FIELD) study, patients with diabetes treated with fenofibrate experienced reductions in the risks of developing microalbuminuria, proliferative retinopathy, and minor amputations.[42,43]

The exact mechanisms whereby statins and fibrates decrease microvascular complications are unknown. Putative mediators include effects on inflammatory cytokines, nitric oxide synthase, endothelial function, and angiogenesis. Diabetic neuropathy is a major risk factor for amputation among patients with diabetes; thus, the reported protective effects of statins and fibrates, if confirmed by randomized controlled trials, could be of tremendous public health significance.

REFERENCES

1. Tornvall P, Walldius D. A comparison between nicotinic acid and acipimox in hypertryglyceridemia—effects on serum lipids, lipoproteins, glucose tolerance and tolerability. *J Intern Med* 1991;230:415–421

2. Garg A, Grundy SM. Nicotinic acid as a therapy for dyslipidemia in non-insulin-dependent diabetes mellitus. *JAMA* 1990;264:723–726

3. Wise A, Foord SM, Fraser NJ, Barnes AA, Elshourbagy N, Eilert M, Ignar DM, Murdock PR, Steplewski K, Green A, Brown AJ, Dowell SJ, Szekeres PG, Hassall DG, Marshall FH, Wilson S, Pike NB. Molecular identification of high and low affinity receptors for nicotinic acid. *J Biol Chem* 2003;278:9869–9874

4. Tunaru S, Kero J, Schaub A, Wufka C, Blaukat A, Pfeffer K, Offermanns S. PUMA-G and HM74 are receptors for nicotinic acid and mediate its antilipolytic effect. *Nat Med* 2003;9:352–355

5. Karpe F, Frayn KN. The nicotinic acid receptor—a new mechanism for an old drug. *Lancet* 2004;363:1892–1894

6. Kamanna VS, Vo A, Kashyap ML. Nicotinic acid: recent developments. *Curr Opin Cardiol* 2008;23:393–398

7. Ganji SH, Tavintharan S, Zhu D, Xing Y, Kamanna VS, Kashyap ML. Niacin noncompetitively inhibits DGAT2 but not DGAT1 activity in HepG2 cells. *J Lipid Res* 2004;45:1835–1845

8. Kamanna VS, Kashyap ML. Mechanism of action of niacin. *Am J Cardiol* 2008;101:20B–26B

9. Balasse EO, Neef MA. Influence of nicotinic acid on the rates of turnover and oxidation of plasma glucose in man. *Metab Clin Exp* 1973;22:1193–1204

10. Thiebaud D, DeFronzo RA, Jacot E, et al. Effect of long chain triglyceride infusion on glucose metabolism in man. *Metab Clin Exp* 1982;31:1128–1136

11. O'Byrne S, Feely J. Effects of drugs on glucose tolerance in non-insulin dependent diabetics (Part II). *Drugs* 1990;40:6–18

12. Poynten AM, Gan SK, Kriketos AD, O'Sullivan A, Kelly JJ, Ellis BA, Chisholm DJ, Campbell LV. Nicotinic acid-induced insulin resistance is related to increased circulating fatty acids and fat oxidation but not muscle lipid content. *Metabolism* 2003;52:699–704

13. McKenney J. New perspectives on the use of niacin in the treatment of lipid disorders. *Arch Intern Med* 2004;164:697–705

14. Blond E, Rieusset J, Alligier M, Lambert-Porcheron S, Bendridi N, Gabert L, Chetiveaux M, Debard C, Chauvin MA, Normand S, Roth H, de Gouville AC, Krempf M, Vidal H, Goudable J, Laville M; "Niacin" Study Group. Nicotinic acid effects on insulin sensitivity and hepatic lipid metabolism: an in vivo to in vitro study. *Horm Metab Res* 2014;46:390–396

15. Henkin Y, Oberman A, Hurst DC, Segrest JP. Niacin revisited: clinical observation on an important but underutilized drug. *Am J Med* 1991;91:239–246

16. Mohan LR, Mohan V. Drug induced diabetes mellitus. *J Assoc Physicians India* 1997;45:876–879

17. Fulcher GR, Jones IR, Alberti KG. Improvement in glucose tolerance by reduction of lipid concentrations in non-insulin dependent diabetes mellitus. *Diabetes News* 1988;9:4–8

18. Grundy SM, Vega GL, McGovern ME, et al. Efficacy, safety and tolerability of once-daily niacin for treatment of dyslipidemia associated with type 2 diabetes. *Arch Intern Med* 2002;162:1568–1573

19. HPS2-THRIVE Collaborative Group. Effects of extended-release niacin with laropiprant in high-risk patients. *N Engl J Med* 2014;371:203–212

20. Ridker PM, Danielson E, Fonseca FAH, Genest J, Gotto AM Jr, Kastelein JJP, Koenig W, Libby P, Lorenzatti AJ, MacFadyen JG, Nordestgaard BG, Shepherd J, Willerson JT, Glynn RJ, for the JUPITER Study Group. Rosuvastatin to prevent vascular events in men and women with elevated C-reactive protein. *N Eng J Med* 2008;359:2195–2207

21. Sasaki J, Iwashita M, Kono S. Statins: beneficial or adverse for glucose metabolism. *J Atheroscler Thromb* 2006;13:123–129

22. Culver AL, Ockene IS, Balasubramanian R, Olendzki BC, Sepavich DM, Wactawski-Wende J, Manson JE, Qiao Y, Liu S, Merriam PA, Rahilly-Tierny C, Thomas F, Berger JS, Ockene JK, Curb JD, Ma Y. Statin use and risk of diabetes mellitus in postmenopausal women in the Women's Health Initiative. *Arch Intern Med* 2012;172:144–152

23. Cederberg H, Stančáková A, Yaluri N, Modi S, Kuusisto J, Laakso M. Increased risk of diabetes with statin treatment is associated with impaired insulin sensitivity and insulin secretion: a 6 year follow-up study of the METSIM cohort [article online]. *Diabetologia* 2015. DOI 10.1007/s00125-015-3528-5

24. Rajpathak SW, Kumbhani DJ, Crandall J, et al. Statin therapy and risk of developing type 2 diabetes: a meta-analysis. *Diabetes Care* 2009;32:1924–1929

25. Jick SS, Bradbury BD. Statins and newly diagnosed diabetes. *Br J Clin Pharmacol* 2004;58:303–309

26. Sattar N, Preiss D, Murray HM, Welsh P, Buckley BM, de Craen AJ, Seshasai SR, McMurray JJ, Freeman DJ, Jukema JW, Macfarlane PW, Packard CJ, Stott DJ, Westendorp RG, Shepherd J, Davis BR, Pressel SL, Marchioli R, Marfisi RM, Maggioni AP, Tavazzi L, Tognoni G, Kjekshus J, Pedersen TR, Cook TJ, Gotto AM, Clearfield MB, Downs JR, Nakamura H, Ohashi Y, Mizuno K, Ray KK, Ford I. Statins and risk of incident diabetes: a collaborative meta-analysis of randomised statin trials. *Lancet* 2010;375:735–742

27. Swerdlow DI, Preiss D, Kuchenbaecker KB, Holmes MV, et al. HMG-coenzyme A reductase inhibition, type 2 diabetes, and bodyweight: evidence from genetic analysis and randomised trials. *Lancet* 2015;385:351–361

28. Nakata M, Nagasaka S, Kusaka I, et al. Effects of statins on the adipocyte maturation and expression of glucose transporter 4. *Diabetologia* 2006;49:1881–1892

29. Yada T, Nakata M, Shiraishi T, et al. Inhibition by simvastatin, but not pravastatin, of glucose-induced cytosolic calcium signaling and insulin secretion due to L-type calcium channels in rat islet β-bells. *Brit J Pharmacol* 1999;126:1205–1213

30. Sattar N, Taskinen. Statins are diabetogenic—myth or reality? *Atherosclerosis Supplements* 2012;13:1–10

31. Erqou S, Lee CC, Adler AI. Statins and glycaemic control in individuals with diabetes: a systematic review and meta-analysis. *Diabetologia* 2014;57:2444–2452

32. U.S. Food and Drug Administration. FDA drug safety communication: important safety label changes to cholesterol lowering statin drugs. 2012.

33. American Diabetes Association. Statement on recent FDA safety changes in labeling for some cholesterol-lowering drugs. 2012

34. Ridker PM, Pradhan A, MacFadyen JG, Libby P, Glynn RJ. Cardiovascular benefits and diabetes risks of statin therapy in primary prevention: an analysis from the JUPITER trial. *Lancet* 2012;380:565–571

35. Diabetes Prevention Program Research Group. Reduction in the incidence of type 2 diabetes with lifestyle intervention or metformin. *N Engl J Med* 2002;346:393–403

36. Flory JH, Ellenberg S, Szapary PO, Strom BL, Hennessy S. Antidiabetic action of bezafibrate in a large observational database. *Diabetes Care* 2009;32:547–551

37. Tenenbaum A, Fisman EZ, Boyko V, Benderly M, Tanne D, Haim M, Matas Z, Motro M, Behar S. Attenuation of progression of insulin resistance in patients with coronary artery disease by bezafibrate. *Arch Intern Med* 2006;166:737–741

38. Tenenbaum A, Motro M, Fisman EZ. Dual and pan-peroxisome proliferator-activated receptors (PPAR) co-agonism: the bezafibrate lessons. *Cardiovasc Diabetol* 2005;4:14

39. Bays HE, Goldberg RB, Truitt KE, Jones MR. Colesevelam hydrochloride therapy in patients with type 2 diabetes mellitus treated with metformin: glucose and lipid effects. *Arch Intern Med* 2008;168:1975–1983

40. Staels B. A review of bile acid sequestrants: potential mechanism(s) for glucose-lowering effects in type 2 diabetes mellitus. *Post Grad Med* 2009;121(3 Suppl. 1):25–30

41. Davis TM, Yeap BB, Davis WA, Bruce DG. Lipid-lowering therapy and peripheral sensory neuropathy in type 2 diabetes: the Fremantle Diabetes Study. *Diabetologia* 2008;51:562–566

42. Keech AC, Mitchell P, Summanen PA, et al., FIELD study investigators. Effect of fenofibrate on the need for laser treatment for diabetic retinopathy (FIELD study): a randomised controlled trial. *Lancet* 2007;370:1687–1697

43. Rajamani K, Colman PG, Li LP, Best JD, Voysey M, D'Emden MC, Laakso M, Baker JR, Keech AC; FIELD study investigators. Effect of fenofibrate on amputation events in people with type 2 diabetes mellitus (FIELD study): a prespecified analysis of a randomised controlled trial. *Lancet* 2009;373:1780–1788

8

Antimicrobial Drugs

ANTIBIOTICS

Emerging evidence indicates that intestinal bacteria, rather than being passive commensals, might be interacting dynamically with metabolic pathways associated with energy balance, obesity, insulin resistance, and diabetes.[1-3] In humans, two groups of bacteria are dominant among gut flora—the Bacteroidetes and the Firmicutes—and there is a decrease in the relative abundance of Bacteroidetes in obese people compared with lean people.[2] Following weight loss, the proportion of beneficial Bacteroidetes is restored to higher levels.[2] To the extent that these changes mirror or reflect complex interactions between gut flora and metabolic pathways linked to the obese phenotype, alterations in native gut flora (such as following antibiotic ingestion) could have implications for the pathogenesis of obesity-related disorders, such as diabetes and cardiovascular disease.

In this regard, a recent report from a large population-based database from the U.K., known as the Health Improvement Network, is strikingly noteworthy.[4] Using a nested case–control design (1 case matched with 4 controls), the authors evaluated the association between antibiotic exposure and diabetes. Cases ($n = 208,002$) were defined as those with incident diagnosis of diabetes, and controls ($n = 815,576$) consisted of all individuals without a diagnosis of diabetes at the date the case was diagnosed. Cases and controls were matched for age, gender, practice site, duration, and calendar period of follow-up. The exposure of interest was antibiotic therapy lasting longer than 1 year before the index date. Using conditional logistic regression, the authors estimated odds ratios and 95% confidence intervals, after adjusting for BMI, smoking, prestudy glucose level, number of infections, and other pertinent factors.[4]

The results showed that exposure to a single antibiotic prescription was not associated with diabetes risk. Treatment with two to five courses of antibiotics, however, was associated with an increased risk of incident diabetes.[4] The adjusted odds ratios ranged from 1.08 (95% CI 1.05–1.11) for penicillin to 1.15 (95% CI 1.08–1.23) for quinolones. The risk of incident diabetes increased with increasing exposure to courses of antibiotic treatment: individuals who received more than five courses of antibiotics showed a 37% increased risk of diabetes (OR 1.37 [95% CI 1.19–1.58]). Although no causality can be confirmed from this case–control study, the results do raise the plausibility that frequent use of certain antibiotics could increase diabetes risk, presumably by decreasing the abundance of beneficial flora or increasing the overgrowth of unfavorable species. With greater insight into the evolving field of gut microbiomics, it may be possible to discover or design antibiotics or probiotics that can shift the balance of gut flora toward metabolically favorable directions.

FLUOROQUINOLONES

Several reports have linked the fluoroquinolone, gatifloxacin (withdrawn from the U.S. market in 2006), to increased risks for dysglycemia (i.e., hyperglycemia or hypoglycemia).[5] Acutely, gatifloxacin stimulates insulin secretion (leading to hypoglycemia), whereas chronic therapy leads to the inhibition of insulin synthesis and secretion.[6,7] The fluoroquinolones share structural similarities with antimalarials (such as quinine, chloroquine, and mefloquine), which are known to stimulate insulin secretion by closing the K_{ATP} channel on pancreatic β-cells.[8] Individual fluoroquinolone antibiotics, however, have differing affinities for the K_{ATP} channel: studies have shown that gatifloxacin and temafloxacin are more avid in this regard than ciprofloxacin and levofloxacin.[9] The risk of dysglycemia does not appear to be a class effect, as currently available quinolones (ciprofloxacin, levofloxacin, and moxifloxacin) have been associated with fewer glucose abnormalities than gatifloxacin.[10] Among outpatients, the frequency of dysglycemic events (number of events divided by total number of treated patients) was 1.1% for gatifloxacin, 0.3% for ciprofloxacin, 0.3% for levofloxacin, and 0.2% for moxifloxacin.[5,11] By contrast, the dysglycemia rate was 0.2% for second-generation cephalosporins and 0.1 % for macrolides.[11] An earlier report among inpatients showed different rates of dysglycemia: gatifloxacin (1.01%), levofloxacin (0.93%), and ciprofloxacin (0%).[12] The complicated illnesses and variable caloric intake among the inpatients make direct comparison with the outpatient rates problematic.

The majority of patients who experience glucose disruption with fluoroquinolones have preexisting diabetes. Hypoglycemia typically occurs within 3 days of drug exposure, but it also has been reported following a single dose. Fluoroquinolone-induced acute insulin secretion can potentiate the effects of concomitant antidiabetic agents and thereby can increase the hypoglycemia risk among patients with diabetes. Overall, hyperglycemia is more prevalent than hypoglycemia in patients treated with quinolones. The mechanism of the hyperglycemia is unclear but likely involves depletion of insulin granules and inhibition of insulin biogenesis, at least in the case of gatifloxacin.[6] Alteration of intestinal flora also is a plausible mechanism for quinolone-associated diabetes.[2,4] Fluoroquinolone-associated hyperglycemia usually presents after several days to weeks of drug exposure. Ambrose et al.[13] have identified renal dysfunction as a major risk factor for hyperglycemia in patients with toxic overdosage with fluoroquinolone.

In a case-control analysis of a large outpatient database (covering 1.4 million patients), the risk of treatment-emergent hyperglycemia was specific to gatifloxacin and was no higher for levofloxacin, moxifloxacin, or ciprofloxacin than other antibiotic classes such as macrolides or cephalosporins.[11] In a smaller chart review study covering ~17,000 inpatients, 92 patients (almost all with preexisting diabetes) had random blood glucose levels of $\geq$200 mg/dL within 3 days of receiving levofloxacin, gatifloxacin, or ceftriaxone.[12] Preexisting diabetes and renal insufficiency were characteristic findings among those who developed fluoroquinolone-associated hyperglycemia.[12] In yet another retrospective analysis, involving >64,000 patients in the Veterans Administration database, use of fluoroquinolones was not associated with hyperglycemia.[14]

These conflicting findings reflect the inherent weakness of the retrospective study design, as compared with randomized controlled trials. Nonetheless, with regard to dysglycemia, the attributes of temporality, biological plausibility, and possibly dose-response have been demonstrated, at least, for one member of the fluoroquinolone family. The incidence of fluoroquinolone-associated glucose abnormalities is low, and the risk appears much lower for agents in current use than for gatifloxacin. Patients with diabetes, the elderly, and those with renal dysfunction should be monitored closely for hyperglycemia (and hypoglycemia) during therapy with fluoroquinolones. Concern over the possible risk of dysglycemia, however, should not override the use of fluoroquinolones for the appropriate indications in patients with or without diabetes.

ANTIRETROVIRAL AGENTS

The use of combination highly active antiretroviral therapy (HAART) has dramatically improved clinical outcomes for people with HIV infection.[15,16] However, adverse metabolic effects, including insulin resistance, diabetes, dyslipidemia, and lipodystrophy,[17] have been associated with HAART. HIV-associated lipodystrophy is characterized by lipoatrophy because of subcutaneous fat loss in the face and lower extremeties and abdominal lipohypertrophy from increased visceral adiposity. These morphological changes are accompanied by insulin resistance, dyslipidemia, and an increased risk for diabetes.[18,19] The clinical presentation of antiretroviral-associated diabetes is consistent with type 2 diabetes, and the underlying mechanisms include insulin resistance and impaired β-cell function. HIV-1 protease inhibitors (PIs) acutely induce insulin resistance and concurrently impair insulin secretion.[20-22] The PIs share structural similarities with glucose transporter (GLUT4; the major intracellular glucose transporter) and probably induce insulin resistance by interfering with glucose transport.[23] In cultured islet cells from an insulinoma cell line, exposure to indinavir and other PIs, such as amprenavir, nelfinavir, and ritonavir, significantly inhibits glucose-stimulated insulin secretion.[24] The risk factors for insulin resistance and diabetes in patients with HIV infection treated with PIs include positive family history of diabetes, weight gain, lipodystrophy, older age, and coinfection with hepatitis C (Table 8.1).[25]

Nucleoside analogs (reverse transcriptase inhibitors) stavudine, zidovudine, and didanosine also are associated with the risk of incident diabetes during long-term follow-up.[26] The increased risk persists after adjustment for diabetes risk factors, which suggests a possible direct effect of the nucleoside analogs on glucoregulation. Indeed, nucleoside analogs have been shown to induce insulin resistance, lipodystrophy, and mitochondrial dysfunction,[27,28] which could be mechanisms for the development of diabetes. In an analysis of 33,389 HIV-infected

Table 8.1—Risk Factors for Diabetes in HIV-Infected Patients

- Family history of diabetes

- Older age

- Medications
  —Protease inhibitors
  —Nucleoside analogs

- Weight gain

- Lipodystrophy

- Co-infection with Hepatitis C

patients, who were followed for incident diabetes, De Wit et al.[26] observed that exposure to stavudine conferred the greatest risk for incident diabetes, compared with other agents, including PIs. The current evidence indicates that PIs confer acute metabolic risks, whereas the nucleoside analogs confer cumulative risk for diabetes over time, and that concurrent exposure to PIs and nucleoside analogs poses additional risk for diabetes among HIV-infected patients.

Physicians who treat patients with HIV-AIDS need to be alert to the adverse metabolic effects of the expanding antiretroviral armamentarium. Furthermore, as a result of the efficacy of HAART and improved nutritional status, many HIV-infected patients in remission experience significant weight gain, which is an additional risk factor for insulin resistance, diabetes, and dyslipidemia.

Approach to Management and Risk Reduction

Lifestyle Modification. The standards of care for diabetes in HIV-infected patients are the same as those for the general diabetes population. The general glycemic goals are as follows: average preprandial capillary plasma glucose values of 80–130 mg/dL, peak postprandial capillary plasma glucose target of <180 mg/dL, and A1C level of 7% or lower.[29] A comprehensive approach incorporating lifestyle modification (diet and exercise) and antidiabetic medications is advocated.[30] Patients with HIV disease and diabetes require an individualized dietary intervention, guided by current weight, state of glycemic control, lipid profile, blood pressure, and presence or absence of catabolic drive from opportunistic infections.

Medications. The approved antidiabetic drugs are effective in controlling hyperglycemia in HIV patients. The potential exists, however, for adverse drug interactions among some of the concomitant medications. Any preexisting hepatic injury (likely from hepatitis C or drug toxicity) precludes the use of thiazolidinediones (TZDs), and patients with HIV nephropathy are not candidates for metformin therapy. Moreover, the gastrointestinal side effects of metformin and α-glucosidase inhibitors (acarbose, miglitol, voglibose) may be limiting in patients with HIV-associated enteropathy. Nucleoside analogs and other agents used in HAART regimens have specific warnings regarding the potential risks of lactic acidosis and severe hepatic dysfunction (Table 8.2).[31] Therefore, close monitoring of liver enzymes is required in patients on HAART who require treatment with TZDs, metformin, or other oral antidiabetic medications. Whenever such complex toxicological considerations exist, exogenous insulin becomes the therapy of choice, but care must be taken regarding needle disposal. Treatment with metreleptin (recombinant human leptin) corrects the metabolic abnormalities associated with lipodystrophy (including insulin resistance, hyperglycemia, hypertriglyceridemia, and hepatic steatosis); initial experience shows efficacy in patients with HIV-associated lipodystrophy.[19,32]

Table 8.2—Antiretroviral Drugs Associated with Lactic Acidosis and Hepatic Dysfunction

Lactic Acidosis/Hepatomegaly	Elevated Transaminases
Nucleoside analogs	**Non-nucleoside RT inhibitors**
–Abacavir	–Delavirdine
–Emtricitabine	–Efavirenz
–Lamivudine	
–Stavudine	**Protease inhibitors**
–Zidovudine	–Fosamprenavir
	–Lopinavir
Nucleoside RT inhibitors	–Ritonavir
–Tenofovir	–Saquinavir

RT—reverse transcriptase. *Source: Physicians' Desk Reference 2015*

Switching. It has been reported anecdotally that switching from PIs to regimens substituted with nevirapine may improve hyperglycemia.[33] Others have suggested that switching from triple regimen to PIs might decrease the risk of lipoatrophy.[34] It generally is not prudent, however, to abruptly discontinue otherwise efficacious antiretroviral agents, and any such decision must be made in consultation with the physicians managing the HIV disease.

REFERENCES

1. Turnbaugh PJ, Ley RE, Mahowald MA, Magrini V, Mardis ER, Gordon JI, Ley RE, Turnbaugh PJ, Klein S, Gordon JI. An obesity-associated gut microbiome with increased capacity for energy harvest. *Nature* 2006;444:1027–1031

2. Ley RE, Turnbaugh PJ, Klein S, Gordon JI. Microbial ecology: human gut microbes associated with obesity. *Nature* 2006;444:1022–1023

3. DiBaise JK, Zhang H, Crowell MD, Krajmalnik-Brown R, Decker GA, Rittmann BE. Gut microbiota and its possible relationship with obesity. *Mayo Clin Proc* 2008;83:460–469

4. Boursi B, Mamtani R, Haynes K, Yang YX. The effect of past antibiotic exposure on diabetes risk. *Eur J Endocrinol* 2015;172:639–648

5. Catero M. Dysglycemia and fluoroquinolones: Are you putting patients at risk? *J Family Prac* 2007;56:101–107

6. Yamada C, Nagashima K, Takahashi A, et al. Gatifloxacin acutely stimulates insulin secretion and chronically suppresses insulin biosynthesis. *Eur J Pharmacol* 2006;553:67–72

7. Tomita T, Onishi M, Sato E, Kimura Y, Kihira K. Gatifloxacin induces augmented insulin release and intracellular insulin depletion of pancreatic islet cells. *Biol Pharm Bull* 2007;30:644–647

8. Gribble FM, Davis TME, Higham CE, Clark A, Ashcroft FM. The antimalarial agent mefloquine inhibits ATP-sensitive K-channels. *Br J Pharmacol* 2000;131:756–760

9. Saraga A, Yokokura M, Gonoi T, et al. Effects of fluoroquinolones on insulin secretion and ß-cell ATP-sensitive K+ channels. *Eur J Pharm* 2004;497:111–117

10. Aspinall SL, Good CB, Jiang R, McCarren M, Dong D, Cunningham FE. Severe dysglycemia with the fluoroquinolones: a class effect? *Clin Infect Dis* 2009;49:402–408

11. Park-Wyllie LY, Juurlink DL, Kopp A, et al. Outpatient gatifloxacin therapy and dysglycemia in older adults. *N Engl J Med* 2006;354:1352–1361

12. Mohr JF, McKinnon PS, Peymann PJ, et al. A retrospective, comparative evaluation of dysglycemias in hospitalized patients receiving gatifloxacin, levofloxacin, ciprofloxacin, or ceftriaxone. *Pharmacother* 2005;25:1303–1309

13. Ambrose PG, Bhavnani SM, Cirincione BB, et al. Gatifloxacin and the elderly: pharmacokinetic-pharmacodynamic rationale for a potential age-related dose reduction. *J Antimicrob Chemother* 2003;S2:434–444

14. Coblio NA, Mowrey K, McCright P, et al. Use of a data warehouse to examine the effect of fluoroquinolones on glucose metabolism. *Am J Health Syst Pharm* 2004;61:2545–2548

15. Palella FJ Jr, Delaney KM, Moorman AC, et al. Declining morbidity and mortality among patients with advanced immunodeficiency virus infection. HIV Outpatient Study Investigators. *N Engl J Med* 1998;338:853–860

16. Dagogo-Jack S. HIV therapy and diabetes risk. *Diabetes Care* 2008;31:1267–1268

17. Dagogo-Jack S. New drugs and diabetes risk: antipsychotic and antiretroviral agents. In *Clinical Diabetes*. Fonseca VA, Ed. Saunders, Philadelphia, 2006, p. 569–581

18. Alves MD, Brites C, Sprinz E. HIV-associated lipodystrophy: a review from a Brazilian perspective. *Ther Clin Risk Manag* 2014;10:559–566

19. Tsoukas MA, Farr OM, Mantzoros CS. Leptin in congenital and HIV-associated lipodystrophy. *Metabolism* 2015;64:47–59

20. Yarasheski KE, Tebas P, Sigmund C, Dagogo-Jack S, Bohrer A, Turk J, Halban P, Cryer PE, Powderly WG. Insulin resistance in HIV protease inhibitor-associated diabetes. *J AIDS* 1999;21:209–216

21. Dube MP, Edmondson-Melancon H, Qian D, Aqeel R, Johnson D, Buchanan TA. Prospective evaluation of the effect of initiating indinavir-based therapy on insulin sensitivity and B-cell function in HIV-infected patients. *J Acquir Immune Defic Syndr* 2001;27:130–134

22. Schütt M, Zhou J, Meier M, Klein HH. Long-term effects of HIV-1 protease inhibitors on insulin secretion and insulin signaling in INS-1 β-cells. *J Endocrinol* 2004;183:445–454

23. Hertel J, Struthers H, Horj CB, Hruz PW. A structural basis for the acute effects of HIV protease inhibitors on GLUT4 intrinsic activity. *J Biol Chem* 2004;279:55147–55152

24. Koster JC, Remedi MS, Qui H, Nichols CG, Hruz PW. HIV protease inhibitors acutely impair glucose-stimulated insulin release. *Diabetes* 2003;52:1695–1700

25. Mehta SH, Moore RD, Thomas DL, Chaisson RE, Sulkowski MS. The effect of HAART and HCV infection on the development of hyperglycemia among HIV-infected persons. *J Acquir Immune Defic Syndr* 2003;33:577–584

26. De Wit S, Sabin CA, Weber R, et al. Incidence and risk factors for new onset diabetes mellitus in HIV infected patients: the D:A:D study. *Diabetes Care* 2008;31:1224–1229

27. Brown TT, Cole SR, Li X, et al. Antiretroviral therapy and the prevalence and incidence of diabetes mellitus in the multicenter AIDS cohort study. *Arch Intern Med* 2005;165:1179–1184

28. Fleischman A, Johnsen S, Systrom DM, et al. Effects of a nucleoside reverse transcriptase inhibitor, stavudine, on glucose disposal and mitochondrial function in muscle of healthy adults. *Am J Physiol Endocrinol Metab* 2007;292:E1666–1673

29. American Diabetes Association. Standards of medical care in diabetes—2015. *Diabetes Care* 2015;38(Suppl. 1):S5–S87

30. Roubenoff R, Weiss L, McDermott A, et al. A pilot study of exercise training to reduce trunk fat in adults with HIV-associated fat redistribution. *AIDS* 1999;13:1373–1375

31. Nerurkar PV1, Pearson L, Frank JE, Yanagihara R, Nerurkar VR. Highly active antiretroviral therapy (HAART)-associated lactic acidosis: in vitro effects of combination of nucleoside analogues and protease inhibitors on mitochondrial function and lactic acid production. *Cell Mol Biol* (Noisy-le-grand) 2003;49:1205–1211

32. Brown RJ, Gorden P. Leptin therapy in patients with lipodystrophy and syndromic insulin resistance. In *Leptin: Regulation and Clinical Applications*. 1st ed. Dagogo-Jack S, Ed. New York, Springer, 2015, p. 225–236

33. Martinez E, Conget I, Lazano L, Casamitjana R, Gatell JM. Reversion of metabolic abnormalities after switching from HIV-1 protease inhibitors to nevirapine. *AIDS* 1999;13:805–810

34. Clumeck N, Hill A, Moecklinghoff C. Effects of switching to protease inhibitor monotherapy on nucleoside analogue-related adverse events. *AIDS Rev* 2014;16:236–245

9

Atypical Antipsychotic and Antidepressant Agents

ATYPICAL ANTIPSYCHOTIC AGENTS

The second-generation or atypical antipsychotic agents (SGAs) improve clinical outcomes and are less likely to induce extrapyramidal side effects, compared with older agents.[1] Their use, however, has been associated with adverse metabolic effects, including diabetes, weight gain, and dyslipidemia. Diabetes has been reported in patients receiving all SGAs in current use.[2] Interestingly, older reports from the last century also associated use of first-generation (typical) antipsychotic agents with the development of diabetes.[3-5] The clinical pattern of antipsychotic associated diabetes (APAD) is consistent with type 2 diabetes (T2D); the mean age at presentation is ~40 years. About two-thirds of patients present with new-onset diabetes, one-third present with exacerbation of preexisting diabetes, and 25% present with diabetic ketoacidosis (DKA) or metabolic acidosis.[6] The frequency of DKA at presentation in patients with APAD is comparable to the 23% rate reported for the general population with T2D.[7]

Putative explanations for treatment-emergent diabetes include preexisting undiagnosed diabetes; increased susceptibility to diabetes resulting from underlying psychiatric disorders;[8,9] a direct drug effect; an indirect effect mediated by weight gain; or an idiosyncratic reaction in susceptible persons that is inherently unpredictable. It must be stressed that a causal link between specific antipsychotic agents and diabetes remains to be proven. The fact that diabetes is reported only in a minority of patients exposed to antipsychotic drugs weakens the case for direct causality. A mechanism driven purely by insulin resistance from antipsychotic-induced weight gain also is unlikely, because compensatory insulin secretion by the β-cells normally restores glucose homeostasis.[10,11] Indeed, most of the Hill's criteria for causality have not been met with regard to the association between antipsychotic drug exposure and incident diabetes, because of paucity of data from randomized controlled studies, inconsistencies in the literature, incomplete documentation of baseline glycemic status, and lack of mechanistic insight, among other reasons.[2,6]

The Clinical Antipsychotic Trials of Intervention Effectiveness (CATIE) was a National Institutes of Health–funded prospective study that documented metabolic data in 1,460 patients with schizophrenia randomized to treatment with four atypical antipsychotic agents (olanzapine, risperidone, quetiapine, ziprasidone) and perphenazine (a typical antipsychotic agent). The primary aim of CATIE was

DOI: 10.2337/9781580406192.09

to compare the overall effectiveness of the five different treatments on clinical outcome of schizophrenia during a mean follow-up of 18 months.[12] Aripiprazole, which was approved by the U.S. Food and Drug Administration (FDA) in 2002, was not formally tested in CATIE.

Approximately 11% of the patients in CATIE had preexisting diabetes, and the proportions were fairly evenly distributed across the drug treatment groups. The CATIE study did not report the frequency of new treatment-emergent cases of diabetes, but the investigators reported the numbers (and percentages) of people who required new added medications for diabetes, as follows: olanzapine 12 (4%), quetiapine 7 (2%), risperidone 8 (2%), perphenazine 5 (2%), and ziprasidone 4 (2%). These rates were not significantly different from each other. Table 9.1 shows the changes in HbA_{1c} and weight during a median 18 months of follow-up of patients in the CATIE study.

Table 9.1 — Weight and HbA_{1c} during Treatment with Antipsychotic Agents

Antipsychotics	Change in HbA1c (%)	Change in Weight (lb)
Olanzapine	0.40±0.07	9.4±0.9
Quetiapine	0.04±0.08	1.1±0.9
Risperidone	0.07±0.08	0.8±0.9
Ziprasidone	0.11±0.09	-1.6±1.1
Perphenazine	0.09±0.09	-2.01±1.1

Source: Lieberman et al.[12]

Thus, the landmark prospective, randomized study, CATIE, showed that chronic treatment with different antipsychotic agents was associated with differential weight gain and changes in glucose levels. The changes in weight, however, were not strictly predictive of treatment-emergent diabetes, the rate of which was modest (~2–4%) and comparable across the antipsychotic agents studied in CATIE, whether typical or antipsychotic.[12] Thus, although weight gain is a general risk factor for T2D, other contributory factors probably interact with adiposity to trigger diabetes in a given individual.[2]

Since completion of the publicly funded CATIE, additional SGAs have been approved for use in the U.S. or elsewhere. These agents along with their FDA approval years (in parentheses) include paliperidone (2006), iloperidone (2009), asenapine (2009), lurasidone (2010), and brexpiprazole (2015). Sertindole and blonanserin are approved and in use for treatment of schizophrenia in countries outside the U.S.[13] Aripiprazole, which was approved by the FDA in 2002, was not formally tested in CATIE. Limited clinical trials data suggest variable effects on weight gain, blood glucose, and lipid profile during short- and long-term exposure to aripiprazole and the newer agents.[14] In general, the direction of the treatment-emergent metabolic changes with these agents tends to be modestly less favorable than placebo (with the exception of lurasidone, which is associated with a slight increase in HDL cholesterol level).[15]

Thus, the expectation that one or more of these newer agents would overall be associated with less adverse metabolic effects than the preexisting SGAs remains to be demonstrated in randomized controlled trials.[14,15]

Approach to Management and Risk Reduction

Monitoring. The risks of suicide, homicide, and other serious harm to self and society in people with psychotic illness mandate that effective control of psychosis remain the top priority. Therefore, physicians should utilize agents that best accomplish that goal, based on proven efficacy and effectiveness data.[12] As recommended by the FDA and the American Diabetes Association Consensus Panel, screening for diabetes risk factors and documentation of baseline glucose levels, weight, waist circumference, BMI, blood pressure, and lipid profile should precede initiation of antipsychotic therapy.[16] The fasting plasma glucose and lipid levels should be repeated after 12 weeks of initiation of antipsychotic therapy, and annually thereafter (Table 9.2).

Table 9.2—American Diabetes Association Screening Guidelines for Patients with SGAs

	Baseline	4 wk	8 wk	12 wk	12 mo	5 yr
Personal/Family History	X					
Weight (BMI)	X	X	X			
Waist circumference	X					
Blood pressure	X					
Fasting glucose	X			X	X	
Fasting lipids	X			X		X

Source: American Diabetes Association[16]
SGA—second-generation antipsychotic

Education and Lifestyle Modification. Patients and their families should be educated regarding the metabolic risks associated with antipsychotic agents.[17] Body weight should be recorded at baseline and every 4 weeks during the first 3 months of treatment with SGAs.[16] Patients with rapid weight gain ($\geq$4 lb during the first month of drug exposure) should receive prompt lifestyle intervention to reverse or limit weight gain. Caloric reduction, food portion control, substitution of beverages with water or sugar-free alternatives, increased physical activity, and close and frequent monitoring of weight and food intake are some of the proven strategies for prevention of antipsychotic-induced weight gain.[18,19] Patients with preexisting diabetes should be monitored for possible glycemic exacerbation, and appropriate adjustments to antidiabetic regimens should be implemented.

Medications. The actual goals and interventions for control of diabetes in patients receiving antipsychotic drugs are similar to those of the general populace. The approved antidiabetic agents retain their efficacy in psychiatric patients, and no adverse interactions with SGAs have been reported. Agents that promote weight loss or are weight neutral may be preferable as initial therapy in obese patients, but most patients eventually require multiple medications for effective glycemic control. Insulin is indicated for severe hyperglycemia, DKA, and hyperosmolar crisis, and for patients whose diabetes is inadequately controlled on oral agents.

Switching

Routine withdrawal of an otherwise effective SGA is imprudent, because of the risk of psychotic relapse. Drug substitution may be compelling under certain circumstances (e.g., severe hyperglycemia, DKA, diabetic coma), but this must be undertaken in close consultation with a psychiatrist. Any drug substitution would be on an empirical basis, as currently no scientific data on differential diabetes risks among individual SGAs are available to guide such practice.

ANTIDEPRESSANTS

Depression as well as use of antidepressant medications has been associated with increased risk for diabetes.[20–22] The exact nature of the relationship between antidepressant medications and diabetes risk is unclear. Tricyclic antidepressants (TCA) have been associated with weight gain[23,24] and worsening glycemia in diabetic patients.[25] However, selective serotonin reuptake inhibitors (SSRIs) and other antidepressants are largely weight neutral; some have even been associated with weight loss and improved insulin sensitivity.[26] Notably, depression occurs more frequently among people with diabetes than the general population[27] and is associated with worse outcome (more diabetic complications, increased mortality).[28,29] Activation of the hypothalamic-pituitary-adrenal axis with resultant hypercortisolemia is a well-known mechanism in depression and major psychiatric disorders.[30] Thus, endogenous steroid-induced dysglycemia could be a factor linking depression to diabetes risk. Indeed, pathological states of hypercortisolemia (such as Cushing's syndrome) often present with depression and dysglycemia, both of which abate following successful correction of the underlying hypercortisolemia.[31]

The Diabetes Prevention Program (DPP) tracked 3,000 subjects with prediabetes (randomized to treatment with lifestyle intervention, metformin, or placebo) for incident T2D during 2.8 years of follow-up. At baseline, 0.3% of DPP participants had symptoms of depression (Beck Depression Index, BDI scores >11) and 5.7% of these were taking antidepressants.[32] Subjects with elevated BDI scores at baseline and those who ever had elevated BDI scores during the DPP were identified. Cox proportional hazard models then were used to evaluate whether elevated depression symptoms or use of antidepressants predicted progression from prediabetes to T2D. After controlling for multiple predictors of diabetes risk (age, gender, fasting glucose, weight change, and ethnicity), elevated BDI scores at baseline or during the DPP study did not predict diabetes risk in any treatment arm. By contrast, use of antidepressant at baseline more than doubled the risk of incident diabetes among participants in the placebo (HR 2.25 [95% CI 1.38–3.66]) and lifestyle (HR 3.48 [95% CI 1.93–6.28]) arms.[32] A follow-up report from the DPP Outcomes Study made the same observation: continuous antidepressant use compared with no use was associated with diabetes risk in the placebo (adjusted HR 2.34 [95% CI 1.32–4.15]) and lifestyle (adjusted HR 2.48 [95% CI 1.45–4.22]) arms.[33] Interestingly, subjects in the metformin arm did not show a relationship between antidepressant use and diabetes risk.

The association between antidepressant use and increased risk of developing T2D in the DPP was seen across all drug classes, including SSRIs and selective serotonin and norepinephrine reuptake inhibitors. The DPP findings are consistent with recent data from a nested case-control study in a cohort of 165,958 patients with depression in the U.K. General Practice Research Database.[22] The U.K. data showed increased diabetes rates for people receiving long-term (>24 months) treatment with moderate to high daily doses of tricyclic antidepressants (TCAs) (incidence rate ratio = 1.77 [95% CI 1.21–2.59]) and SSRI (incidence rate ratio = 2.06 [95% CI 1.20–3.52]). No increase in diabetes risk was observed for shorter courses or lower daily doses of antidepressants. Another study reported higher risk of diabetes for people receiving combined treatment with SSRIs and TCAs than those treated with TCAs alone.[34]

The exact mechanism(s) for the reported increased risk of diabetes from antidepressants are unclear; the weight gain sometimes associated with TCA use is not sufficient explanation for the development of diabetes. In the DPP, use of antidepressants predicted increased diabetes risk after controlling for weight gain. Moreover, in the DPP, the predominant antidepressants used were SSRIs and related agents, medications generally considered to be weight neutral or even associated with weight loss. One plausible explanation is that antidepressant use probably reflects severe or chronic depression, which has a stronger association with diabetes risk than mild depression.[33,35,36]

Approach to Risk Reduction

Until the exact mechanisms are elucidated, it is prudent to screen for diabetes at baseline and monitor blood glucose levels at reasonable intervals during treatment with all antidepressants. It is equally important to recognize and treat occult depression in patients with diabetes, as the prevalence has been estimated to be as high as 20–25%.[37–39] Comorbid depression is associated with increased mortality in people with diabetes, and must be diagnosed and treated promptly.[29] Although there is a variable potential risk of worsening of glycemic control during antidepressant therapy (Lustman et al., 1997; Lustman et al., 2000; Kammer et al., 2015), that concern should not prevent the appropriate use of antidepressants in patients with diabetes and depression.[25,40,41] If glycemic deterioration occurs during antidepressant therapy in a patient with diabetes, the concomitant antidiabetes regimen can be optimized to achieve improved control.

In people who do not have diabetes, the emerging data suggest that treatment with lower doses of antidepressants and for a shorter duration (< 24 months) may be associated with a lower risk of incident diabetes. Therefore, whenever clinically feasible, clinicians should aim to minimize the dose and duration of antidepressant therapy, without jeopardizing the overall mental health of the patient. People with risk factors for diabetes (Table 1.1) who require long-term antidepressant therapy should receive lifestyle counseling for diabetes prevention (Table 9.1)[42,43] on empirical grounds. Although the DPP showed that metformin treatment was associated with apparent protection from antidepressant-associated diabetes,[32] further studies are needed before metformin prophylaxis can be recommended routinely. Metformin, however, may be considered on empirical grounds in high-risk patients who develop treatment-emergent prediabetes or dysglycemia during prolonged antidepressant therapy. The latter would be consistent with the general recommendation by an Expert Panel of the American Diabetes Association regarding selective use of metformin in prediabetes.[44]

REFERENCES

1. Freedman R. Schizophrenia. *N Eng J Med* 2003;349:1738–1749

2. Dagogo-Jack S. The role of antipsychotic agents in the development of diabetes. *Nat Clin Pract Endocrinol Metab* 2009;5:22–23

3. Meduna LJ, Gerty FJ, Urse VG. Biochemical disturbances in mental disorders. *Arch Gen Psychiatry* 1942;47:38–52

4. Thonnard-Neumann E. Phenothiazines and diabetes in hospitalized women. *Am J Psychiatry* 1968;124:138–142

5. Keskiner A, el Toumi A, Bousquet T. Psychotropic drugs, diabetes and chronic mental patients. *Psychosomatics* 1973;14:176–181

6. Dagogo-Jack S. New drugs and diabetes risk: antipsychotic and antiretroviral agents. In *Clinical Diabetes*. Fonseca VA, Ed. Saunders, Philadelphia, 2006, p. 569–581

7. Johnson DD, Palumbo PJ, Chu CP. Diabetic ketoacidosis in a community-based population. *Mayo Clin Proc* 1980;55:83–88

8. Dixon L, Weiden PJ, Delahanty J, et al. Prevalence and correlates of diabetes in national schizophrenia samples. *Schizophr Bull* 2000;26:903–912

9. Fernandez-Egea E, Bernardo M, Parellada E, Justicia A, Garcia-Rizo C, Esmatjes E, Conget I, Kirkpatrick B. Glucose abnormalities in the siblings of people with schizophrenia. *Schizophr Res* 2008;103:110–113

10. Polonsky KS, Sturis J, Bell GI. Non-insulin-dependent diabetes mellitus—a genetically programmed failure of the β cell to compensate for insulin resistance. *N Engl J Med* 1996;334:777–783

11. Sowell MO, Mukhopadhyay N, Cavazzoni P, et al. Hyperglycemic clamp assessment of insulin secretory responses in normal subjects treated with olanzapine, risperidone, or placebo. *J Clin Endocrinol Metab* 2002; 87:2918–2923

12. Lieberman JA, Stroup TS, McEvoy JP, Swartz MS, Rosenheck RA, Perkins DO, Keefe RS, Davis SM, Davis CE, Lebowitz BD, Severe J, Hsiao JK; Clinical Antipsychotic Trials of Intervention Effectiveness (CATIE) Investigators. Effectiveness of antipsychotic drugs in patients with chronic schizophrenia. *N Engl J Med* 2005;353:1209–1223

13. Wang SM, Han C, Lee SJ, Patkar AA, Masand PS, Pae CU. Asenapine, blonanserin, iloperidone, lurasidone, and sertindole: distinctive clinical characteristics of 5 novel atypical antipsychotics. *Clin Neuropharmacol* 2013;36:223–238

14. De Hert M, Detraux J, van Winkel R, Yu W, Correll CU. Metabolic and cardiovascular adverse effects associated with antipsychotic drugs. *Nat Rev Endocrinol* 2011;8:114–126

15. De Hert M, Yu W, Detraux J, et al. Body weight and metabolic adverse effects of asenapine, iloperidone, lurasidone and paliperidone in the treatment of schizophrenia and bipolar disorder: a systematic review and exploratory meta-analysis. *CNS Drugs* 2012;26:733–759

16. American Diabetes Association. Consensus Development Conference on antipsychotic drugs and obesity and diabetes. *Diabetes Care* 2004;27:596–601

17. Keck PE Jr, Buse JB, Dagogo-Jack S, et al. Managing metabolic concerns in patients with severe mental illness: a special report. *Postgrad Med*, Minneapolis, MN, McGraw-Hill;2003, 1–92

18. Menza M, Vreeland B, Minsky S, et al. Managing atypical antipsychotic-associated weight gain: 12-month data on a multimodal weight control program. *J Clin Psychiatry* 2004;65:471–477

19. Hoffmann VP, Ahl J, Meyers A, et al. Wellness intervention for patients with serious and persistent mental illness. *J Clin Psychiatry* 2005;66:1576–1579

20. Eaton WW, Armenian H, Gallo J, Pratt L, Ford DE. Depression and risk for onset of type II diabetes. A prospective population-based study. *Diabetes Care* 1996;19:1097–1102

21. Knol MJ, Twisk JWR, Beekman ATF, Heine RJ, Snoek FJ, Pouwer F. Depression as a risk factor for the onset of type 2 diabetes: a meta-analysis. *Diabetologia* 2006;49:837–845

22. Andersohn F, Schade R, Suissa S, Garbe E. Long-term use of antidepressants for depressive disorders and the risk of diabetes mellitus. *Am J Psychiatry* 2009;166:591–598

23. Fava M. Weight gain and antidepressants. *J Clin Psychiatry* 2000;61(Suppl. 11):37-41

24. Aronne LJ, Segal KR. Weight gain in the treatment of mood disorders. *J Clin Psychiatry* 2003;64:22–29

25. Lustman PJ, Griffith LS, Clouse RE, Freedland KE, Eisen SA, Rubin EH, Carney RM, McGill JB. Effects of nortriptyline on depression and glycemic control in diabetes: results of a double-blind, placebo controlled trial. *Psychosom Med* 1997;59:241–250

26. Maheux P, Ducros F, Bourque J, Garon J, Chiasson J-L. Fluoxetine improves insulin sensitivity in obese patients with non-insulin-dependent diabetes mellitus independent of weight loss. *Int J Obes Relat Metab Disord* 1997;21:97–102

27. Egede LE, Zheng D. Independent factors associated with major depressive disorder in a national sample. *Diabetes Care* 2003;26:104–111

28. de Groot M, Anderson R, Freedland KE, Clouse RE, Lustman PJ. Association of depression and diabetes complications: a meta-analysis. *Psychosom Med* 2001;63:619–630

29. Katon WJ, Rutter C, Simon G, Lin EHB, Ludman E, Chiechanowski P, Kinder L, Young B, Von Korff M. The association of comorbid depression with mortality in patients with type 2 diabetes. *Diabetes Care* 2005;28:2668–2672

30. Yehuda R, Boisoneau D, Mason JW, Giller EL. Glucocorticoid receptor number and cortisol excretion in mood, anxiety, and psychotic disorders. *Biol Psychiatry* 1993;34:18–25

31. Welbourn RB, Montgomery DA, Kennedy TL. The natural history of treated Cushing's syndrome. *Br J Surg* 1971;58:1–16

32. Diabetes Prevention Program Research Group. Elevated depression symptoms, antidepressant medicine use and risk of developing diabetes during the Diabetes Prevention Program. *Diabetes Care* 2008;31:420–426

33. Rubin RR, Ma Y, Peyrot M, Marrero DG, Price DW, Barrett-Connor E, Knowler WC; Diabetes Prevention Program Research Group. Antidepressant medicine use and risk of developing diabetes during the Diabetes Prevention Program and Diabetes Prevention Program Outcomes study. *Diabetes Care* 2010;33:2549–2551

34. Brown LC, Majumdar SR, Johnson JA. Type of antidepressant therapy and risk of type 2 diabetes in people with depression. *Diabetes Res Clin Pract* 2008;79:61–67

35. Palinkas LA, Barrett-Connor E, Wingard DL. Type 2 diabetes and depressive symptoms in older adults: a population-based study. *Diabet Med* 1991;8:532–539

36. Wing RR, Marcus MD, Blair EH, Epstein LH, Burton LR. Depressive symptomatology in obese adults with type II diabetes. *Diabetes Care* 1990;13:170–172

37. Bot M, Pouwer F, Zuidersma M, van Melle JP, de Jonge P. Association of coexisting diabetes and depression with mortality after myocardial infarction. *Diabetes Care* 2012;35:503–509

38. Chen P-C, Chan Y-T, Chen H-F, Ko M-C, Li C-Y. Population-based cohort analyses of the bidirectional relationship between type 2 diabetes and depression. *Diabetes Care* 2013;36:376–382

39. American Diabetes Association. Standards of medical care in diabetes—2015. *Diabetes Care* 2015;38(Suppl. 1):S5–S87

40. Lustman PJ, Freedland KE, Griffith LS, Clouse RE. Fluoxetine for depression in diabetes: a randomized, double-blind, placebo-controlled trial. *Diabetes Care* 2000;23:618-623

41. Kammer JR, Hosler AS, Leckman-Westin E, DiRienzo G, Osborn CY. The association between antidepressant use and glycemic control in the Southern Community Cohort Study (SCCS). *J Diabetes Complications* 2015 Nov 11. pii: S1056-8727(15)00436-5. doi: 10.1016/j.jdiacomp.2015.10.017 [Epub ahead of print]

42. Diabetes Prevention Program Research Group. Reduction in the incidence of type 2 diabetes with lifestyle intervention or metformin. *N Engl J Med* 2002;346:393–403

43. Dagogo-Jack S. Lifestyle intervention to reduce metabolic and cardiovascular risks. In *Therapeutic Strategies in Metabolic Syndrome*. Fonseca V, Ed. Oxford, Atlas Medical Publishing, 2008, p. 1–19

44. Nathan DM, Davidson MB, DeFronzo RA, et al. Impaired fasting glucose and impaired glucose tolerance: implications for care. *Diabetes Care* 2007;30:753–759

10

Recreational Drugs

ALCOHOL

The relationship between alcohol consumption and diabetes risk is complex. Habitual excessive alcohol intake is a major risk factor for chronic pancreatitis, which is associated with increased diabetes risk. In one longitudinal study that evaluated 656 patients with chronic pancreatitis, the cumulative rate of diabetes over an 8-year period was 50.4%.[1] Alcoholic pancreatitis accounted for two-thirds of all new diabetes cases, and continuous alcoholic intake aggravated chronic pancreatitis and increased the risk of diabetes in the study cohort.[1] Furthermore, in patients with established diabetes, alcohol consumption is associated with adverse effects, including increased risk of hypoglycemia, delayed recovery from hypoglycemia, impaired cognitive and self-management skills, and exacerbation of neuropathic pain.[2-5]

In contrast, the metabolic benefits of moderate alcohol intake have been known for many years.[6-8] In the Diabetes Prevention Program, subjects who reported moderate alcohol intake ($\geq$1 drink/day) had higher high-density lipoprotein (HDL) cholesterol levels and lower incidence rates of diabetes compared with those who consumed less or no alcohol.[9] After adjustment for age, sex, ethnicity, weight, exercise, calorie intake, insulin resistance, insulin secretion, fasting plasma glucose, and weight over time, moderate alcohol consumption was associated with ~40% decrease in diabetes risk compared with nondrinkers.[9] The beneficial effects of moderate alcohol intake were confined to subjects randomized to the lifestyle intervention or metformin therapy, but not placebo, arm of the study.[9] Thus, at least in the Diabetes Prevention Program (a study that enrolled high-risk people with prediabetes), alcohol seemed to augment the beneficial effects of dietary modification and increased physical activity, or concurrent therapy with metformin.

The mechanisms by which moderate alcohol consumption appears to reduce diabetes risk have not been fully explored.[10] Owing to the risks of hypoglycemia and other adverse effects, the American Diabetes Association cautions that patients with diabetes should avoid excessive alcohol consumption (no more than two drinks per day in men and no more than one drink per day in women).[11]

NICOTINE

Diabetic patients with a current history of cigarette smoking tend to have higher HbA_{1c} and lipoprotein levels compared with nonsmokers.[12] Cigarette smoking also is associated with the metabolic syndrome,[13] and new-onset diabetes.[14] The mechanisms for the association between smoking and dysglycemia include induction of insulin resistance, increased hepatic lipase activity, chronic elevation of stress hormones, endothelial dysfunction, and vasoconstrictive effect of nicotine.[15–17]

The return of blood pressure, heart rate, and blood flow and skin temperature of hands and feet to normal within 20 min after smoking cessation indicates rapid reversibility of the acute vasoconstrictive effects of nicotine. Rigorous intervention studies testing the effect of smoking cessation on dysglycemia or incident diabetes are yet to be reported. Nonetheless, there are compelling reasons to promote smoking cessation among diabetic and diabetes-prone subjects: these include the expected pulmonary, cardiovascular, cerebrovascular, and mortality benefits that accompany smoking cessation.[18] Current approaches include cognitive behavioral therapy, use of tapered transdermal or buccal nicotine, and prescription medications (bupropion, varenicline) to decrease craving during the transitional period.[19,20]

MARIJUANA AND CANNABINOIDS

The well-known effects of cannabinoids on appetite stimulation and food intake[21–23] would predict that chronic use could result in weight gain and increase the risk for dysglycemia. This notion is strengthened by recent data showing weight reduction and improvement in glycemic control, following treatment with the endocannabinoid receptor blocker, rimonabant.[24] Yet, paradoxically, marijuana use has been associated with lower BMI[22,25] and lower prevalence of obesity.[26] Penner et al.[25] analyzed a U.S. national cross-sectional sample of 4,657 adults (including 579 current marijuana users and 1,975 past users) who participated in the National Health and Nutrition Examination Survey (NHANES) from 2005 to 2010. Compared with nonusers, current marijuana users had lower values for BMI, waist circumference, fasting glucose and fasting insulin, and less insulin resistance (as estimated by homeostasis model assessment).[25] Reports on the relationship between marijuana use and BMI have been discordant. Among young adults, no significant association between use of marijuana and BMI was seen,[23] but an inverse association between marijuana use and obesity was observed in large U.S. national surveys.[22,26] The National Health and Nutrition Examination Survey (NHANES) III data also showed a lower prevalence of diabetes among marijuana users.[27]

The mechanisms underlying the seemingly paradoxical metabolic associations of marijuana use have not been determined. Also unknown are the effects of chronic marijuana use on long-term cardiometabolic risk factors and clinical outcomes. The extant descriptive studies do not proffer any mechanisms that might explain a link between marijuana use and lower BMI and decreased diabetes risk. Treatment with one of the active ingredients of marijuana, cannabidiol, has been reported to decrease weight in a rodent model.[28] There is evidence that plant cannabinoids act as partial agonists at both the cannabinoid (CB) type 1 and 2 receptors, whereas cannabidiol (which has lower affinity for the CB receptors) appears to antagonize both CB 1 and CB2 receptors.[29,30] Moreover, repeated administration of cannabinoids can decrease the expression of CB1 receptors,[29,31] and cannabinoid receptor knockout mice have a lean phenotype and are resistant to diet-induced obesity.[32] Studies using the CB1 receptor antagonist, rimonabant, offer insights into the metabolic effects of chronic inhibition of CB receptors. Improved insulin sensitivity was noted following treatment with rimonabant in wild-type mice.[33] However, the same treatment was without effect in mice with targeted deletion of the adiponectin gene, a finding that suggests a mediating role for adiponectin in the improvement in insulin sensitivity following inhibition of CB1.[33,34]

As noted at the beginning of this section, human studies have confirmed a wide range of metabolic benefits (including weight loss, decreased waist circumference, improved lipids and insulin sensitivity, and increased adiponectin) following treatment with the CB1 antagonist rimonabant.[24,35,36] Thus, theoretically, an association between marijuana use and lower BMI and waist circumference could occur if the active phytocannabinoid ingredients chronically exert an antagonistic effect on CB1 receptors to produce rimonabant-like metabolic effects in humans. This notion needs to be demonstrated, however, as primary mechanistic data from humans are lacking. Also, although lower adiposity and improved insulin sensitivity could explain decreased risk for diabetes, further studies are needed to understand the impact of chronic marijuana use on incident diabetes and cardiometabolic outcomes in humans. Given these uncertainties, and its adverse neuropsychiatric effects,[37–40] there is currently no scientific rationale for considering marijuana as a possible intervention for managing obesity or decreasing diabetes risk.

OPIOIDS

Historically, a phenomenological connection between diabetes and endogenous opioids was recognized when increased sensitivity to endogenous opioids was identified as the basis of the curious chlorpropamide alcohol flushing.[41] Research evidence accrued since the 1980s suggest that endogenous opioids may be involved in the modulation of glucoregulatory mechanisms, such as insulin secretion and insulin action.[42,43] For example, opioids have been shown to have a deleterious effect on insulin secretion, and the opioid antagonist naloxone briskly augments glucose-stimulated insulin secretion in patients with type 2 diabetes.[42,44–46] Opioid receptors are expressed in skeletal muscles, and β-endorphin has been shown to stimulate the uptake of 2-deoxy-D-[1-3H] glucose, into isolated soleus muscles of lean and obese-diabetic (ob/ob) mice.[47] Increased opioid receptor density was noted in obese-diabetic mice, which suggests an adaptive response.[47] Female mice treated chronically with oral methadone for 35 days experienced hyperglycemia and decreased glycolytic enzyme activity, a phenotype akin to insulin-resistant diabetes.[48]

Treatment of obese subjects with the opioid antagonist naloxone inhibited the insulin and C-peptide responses to glucose administration, suggesting that endogenous β-endorphins increase the responsiveness of the pancreatic β-cells and that opioid administration may contribute to the hyperinsulinemia and the hyperphagia of obesity.[42,44-46,49] In contrast, in obese women, naltrexone decreased basal concentration of both insulin and C-peptide, but did not affect the insulin secretory response to an oral glucose tolerance test.[49] Interestingly, obese women treated with naloxone showed more significant weight loss than obese men,[49] which may be linked to a sex-related difference in opioid effects.

Opioid mechanisms also modulate food intake.[49-51] The effect of opioids on food intake could result in hyperphagia or anorexia, depending on the dose and species of opioids.[49-51] On balance, most studies in rodents indicate that central administration of opioid peptides from three families (endorphins, enkephalins, and dynorphins) increases food intake, and opioid antagonists decrease food intake.[50-52] Chronic opiate use also induces hypogonadism,[49] which is an additional mechanism for increased body fat accumulation and insulin resistance.

These biological effects are likely to carry over to humans: significant weight loss has been documented in humans treated with the opiate antagonist naloxone,[53] and an extended-release formulation of the opioid antagonist naltrexone, in combination with bupropion, recently has been approved by the U.S. Food and Drug Administration for antiobesity therapy.[54] At the clinical level, a phenotype characterized by insulin resistance, elevated HbA_{1c} levels, and markedly decreased acute insulin secretory response to i.v. glucose (but not to arginine) has been described among heroin addicts.[43,55,56] Together with opioid-associated obesity and hypogonadism, the overall phenotype appears to be diabetogenic. Opioids and opioid peptides probably act centrally through the sympathetic nervous system to exert their dysmetabolic and hyperglycemic effects.[42] Thus, opioid addiction is associated with insulin resistance and impaired glucose sensing by the pancreatic β-cells. These metabolic effects, and the consequent potential diabetes risk, have public health significance because opioid abuse has been on the increase, from increased access to prescription opioids, increasing use of opioids for noncancer chronic pain, and escalating illicit use. Surveys of incident diabetes among opiate addicts are scant, and the true impact on diabetes and cardiometabolic disorders remains to be quantified.

In contrast to the foregoing discussion of the hyperglycemic potential of opioids, there have been reports that tramadol, a weak opioid analgesic, actually might be associated with an increased risk of hypoglycemia.[57,58] In a nested case-control database analysis from the U.K., which included 334,034 patients (of whom 1,105 were hospitalized for hypoglycemia), exposure to tramadol was associated with an increased risk of hospitalization for hypoglycemia (~50% higher than the comparator drug, codeine).[58] The risk of hypoglycemia was particularly high during the initial 30 days of exposure to tramadol (OR 2.61 [95% CI 1.61–4.23]).[58] The actual incidence of hospitalization for hypoglycemia was low (8 events per >26,000 person-months of tramadol therapy). Unreported less severe hypoglycemic episodes probably occurred much more frequently, however, and likely were attributed to other causes in patients with or without diabetes who also were receiving treatment with tramadol. Given the increasing use of tramadol as an analgesic for somatic and neuropathic pain in the general population,[59] the association with the risk of hypoglycemia (including severe episodes requiring hospitalization) is noteworthy. An increased awareness of the risk of hypoglycemia is particularly warranted when managing patients with painful diabetic neuropathy who require palliation with agents like tramadol.

Human-level data are unavailable to determine the mechanism of tramadol-associated hypoglycemia. Tramadol has low affinity for opioid receptors but inhibits the neuronal reuptake of serotonin and norepinephrine, which is the mechanism thought to mediate its analgesic effects. Documented effects of tramadol in rodents include inhibition of hepatic gluconeogenesis and stimulation of peripheral glucose utilization[60] and augmentation of insulin signaling in the cerebral cortex and hypothalamus.[61] Both of these effects, which can be blocked by naloxone, would increase the risk of hypoglycemia.[62] It is unclear, however, why tramadol is uniquely associated with hypoglycemia, whereas that risk is not seen with similar compounds that act via the same opioid receptors, such as morphine or oxycodone. In fact, as discussed in the preceding section, these other opioids tend to be associated with mechanisms that predict hyperglycemia (e.g., insulin resistance and impaired insulin secretion).

COCAINE, AMPHETAMINE, AND PSYCHOSTIMULANT DRUGS

Date are limited data on the effects of cocaine on diabetes risk. Sporadic reports have associated cocaine use with hyperglycemic crises (including diabetic ketoacidosis and nonketotic hyperosmolar syndrome) in people with preexisting diabetes.[63–65] The potential mechanisms for hyperglycemic crisis include cocaine-induced discharge of counterregulatory hormones, such as catecholamines[66] and glucocorticoids.[67,68] Thus, a history of cocaine abuse in a patient with diabetes should be considered as a risk factor for hyperglycemic crisis; however, further studies are needed to determine whether habitual use of cocaine increases the risk of new-onset diabetes, especially among individuals who harbor demographic, familial, or morphometric risk factors for diabetes.

Besides cocaine, other sympathomimetic drugs (whether used as recreational stimulants or prescribed for specific indications) can trigger increased secretion of norepinephrine and dopamine.[69,70] Norepinephrine inhibits insulin secretion, induces insulin resistance, and exerts a myriad of metabolic and glucoregulatory actions, mediated by α- and β-adrenergic receptors. In adipose tissue, norepinephrine activates $\beta3$-adrenergic receptors, leading to downstream activation of adenylate cyclase and phosphorylation of hormone-sensitive lipase by a cAMP-dependent protein kinase. The activated hormone-sensitive lipase catalyzes the breakdown of stored triglycerides, with the release of nonesterified fatty acids (NEFA) and glycerol into the circulation. Within hepatocytes, the products of lipolysis extracted from the circulation become gluconeogenic precursors, and β-oxidation of NEFA in mitochondria generates the ketogenic precursors, acetoacetate and acetyl-coenzyme A.[71] Such a broad range of metabolic effects can lead to hyperglycemia (sometimes severe) in patients with inadequate endogenous insulin secretory capacity.

The compounds capable of stimulating increased norepinephrine secretion include amphetamine, methamphetamine, dextroamphetamine, methylenedioxy-methamphetamine (MDMA or Ecstasy), and phentermine. Not surprisingly, reports of diabetes ketoacidosis have appeared in connection with exposure to mephedrone (a recreational drug that stimulates the release of dopamine, serotonin, and norepinephrine), diethylpropion (an amphetamine-like prescription weight-loss drug), and other drugs of habit in patients with diabetes.[72,73] What remains unclear is whether the chronic use of amphetamine-like psychoactive stimulants would disrupt glucose regulation and increase the risk of diabetes in people without a history of diabetes. From the foregoing review of the neuroendocrine mechanisms, there is a theoretical possibility that people with genetic predisposition to diabetes could experience accelerated development of diabetes as a result of persistent exposure to the diabetogenic effects of chronic catechlamine secretion, induced by amphetamine-like drugs.

Interestingly, some prescription weight-loss medications (such as phentermine and phentermine/topiramate) belong to the sympathomimetic family. No concern has been raised thus far, however, regarding the risk of drug-induced hyperglycemia from these antiobesity medications.[74] It is possible that any potential risk associated with increased catecholamine tone is counterbalanced (or outweighed) by the beneficial effects of the weight loss induced by these agents. Overall, there is a dearth of information regarding the use of recreational drugs and diabetes risk. Given the widespread drug habit in society and the escalating diabetes epidemic, well-designed studies on exposure to hard drugs and diabetes risk are sorely needed.

REFERENCES

1. Ito T, Otsuki M, Itoi T, Shimosegawa T, Funakoshi A, Shiratori K, Naruse S, Kuroda Y; Research Committee of Intractable Diseases of the Pancreas. Pancreatic diabetes in a follow-up survey of chronic pancreatitis in Japan. *J Gastroenterol* 2007;42:291–297

2. Richardson T, Weiss M, Thomas P, Kerr D. Day after the night before: influence of evening alcohol on risk of hypoglycemia in patients with type 1 diabetes. *Diabetes Care* 2005;28:1801–1802

3. Rasmussen BM, Orskov L, Schmitz O, Hermansen K. Alcohol and glucose counterregulation during acute insulin-induced hypoglycemia in type 2 diabetic subjects. *Metabolism* 2001;50:451–457

4. Cheyne EH, Sherwin RS, Lunt MJ, Cavan DA, Thomas PW, Kerr D. Influence of alcohol on cognitive performance during mild hypoglycaemia: implications for type 1 diabetes. *Diabet Med* 2004;21:230–237

5. Ferrari LF, Levine E, Levine JD. Independent contributions of alcohol and stress axis hormones to painful peripheral neuropathy. *Neuroscience* 2013;228:409–417

6. Hulley SB, Gordon S. Alcohol and high-density lipoprotein cholesterol: causal inference from diverse study designs. *Circulation* 1981;64(Suppl. 3): 57–63

7. Maclure M. Demonstration of deductive meta-analysis: ethanol intake and risk of myocardial infarction. *Epidemiol Rev* 1993;15:328–351

8. Rimm EB, Moats S. Alcohol and coronary heart disease: drinking patterns and mediators of effect. *Ann Epidemiol* 2007;17:S3–S7

9. Crandall JP, Polsky S, Howard AA, et al. Alcohol consumption and diabetes risk in the Diabetes Prevention Program. *Am J Clin Nutr* 2009;90:595–601

10. Albert MA, Glynn RJ, Ridker PM. Alcohol consumption and plasma concentration of C-reactive protein. *Circulation* 2003;107:443–447

11. American Diabetes Association. Standards of medical care in diabetes—2015. *Diabetes Care* 2016;38:S26.

12. Stamler J, Vaccaro O, Neaton JD, et al. Diabetes, other risk factors, and 12-year mortality for men screened in the Multiple Risk Factor Intervention Trial. *Diabetes Care* 1993;16:434–444

13. Miyatake N, Wada J, Kawasaki Y, Nishii K, Makino H, Numata T. Relationship between metabolic syndrome and cigarette smoking in the Japanese population. *Intern Med* 2006;45:1039–1043

14. Mozaffarian D, Kamineni A, Carnethon M, Djoussé L, Mukamal KJ, Siscovick D. Lifestyle risk factors and new-onset diabetes mellitus in older adults: the cardiovascular health study. *Arch Intern Med* 2009;169:798–807

15. Facchini FS, Hollenbeck CB, Jeppesen J, Chen YD, Reaven GM. Insulin resistance and cigarette smoking. *Lancet* 1992;339:1128–1130

16. Heizer T, Yla-Herttuala S, Luoma J, et al. Cigarette smoking potentiates endothelial dysfunction of forearm resistance vessels in patients with hypercholesterolemia: role of oxidized LDL. *Circulation* 1996;9:1346–1353

17. Kong C, Nimmo L, Elatrozy T, et al. Smoking is associated with increased hepatic lipase activity, insulin resistance, dyslipidaemia and early atherosclerosis in type 2 diabetes. *Atherosclerosis* 2001;156:373–378

18. Taylor DH Jr, Hasselblad V, Henley SJ, Thun MJ, Sloan FA. Benefits of smoking cessation for longevity. *Am J Public Health* 2002;92:990–996

19. Prochaska JO, Velicer WF, Prochaska JM, Johnson JL. Size, consistency, and stability of stage effects for smoking cessation. *Addict Behav* 2004;29:207–213

20. Ranney L, Melvin C, Lux L, McClain E, Lohr KN. Systematic review: smoking cessation intervention strategies for adults and adults in special populations. *Ann Intern Med* 2006;145:845–856

21. Foltin RW, Fischman MW, Byrne MF. Effects of smoked marijuana on food intake and body weight of humans living in a residential laboratory. *Appetite* 1988;11:1–14

22. Smit E, Crespo CJ. Dietary intake and nutritional status of US adult marijuana users: results from the Third National Health and Nutrition Examination Survey. *Public Health Nutr* 2001;4:781–786

23. Rodondi N, Pletcher MJ, Liu K, Hulley SB, Sidney S. Marijuana use, diet, body mass index, and cardiovascular risk factors (from the CARDIA study). *Am J Cardiol* 2006;98:478–484

24. Scheen AJ, Finer N, Hollander P, Jensen MD, Van Gaal LF; RIO-Diabetes Study Group. Efficacy and tolerability of rimonabant in overweight or obese patients with type 2 diabetes: a randomised controlled study. *Lancet* 2006;368:1660–1672

25. Penner EA, Buettner H, Mittleman MA. The impact of marijuana use on glucose, insulin, and insulin resistance among US adults. *Am J Med* 2013;126:583–589

26. Le Strat Y, Le Foll B. Obesity and cannabis use: results from 2 representative national surveys. *Am J Epidemiol* 2011;174:929–933

27. Rajavashisth TB, Shaheen M, Norris KC, et al. Decreased prevalence of diabetes in marijuana users: cross-sectional data from the National Health and Nutrition Examination Survey (NHANES) III. *BMJ Open* 2012;2:e000494

28. Weiss L, Zeira M, Reich S, et al. Cannabidiol lowers incidence of diabetes in non-obese diabetic mice. *Autoimmunity* 2006;39:143–151

29. Pertwee RG. The diverse CB1 and CB2 receptor pharmacology of three plant cannabinoids: delta9-tetrahydrocannabinol, cannabidiol and delta9-tetrahydrocannabivarin. *Br J Pharmacol* 2008;153:199–215

30. Petitet F, Jeantaud B, Reibaud M, Imperato A, Dubroeucq M-C. Complex pharmacology of natural cannabinoids: evidence for partial agonist activity of D9-tetrahydrocannabinol and antagonist activity of cannabidiol on rat brain cannabinoid receptors. *Life Sci* 1998;63:PL1–PL6

31. Hirvonen J, Goodwin RS, Li CT, et al. Reversible and regionally selective downregulation of brain cannabinoid CB1 receptors in chronic daily cannabis smokers. *Mol Psychiatry* 2012;17:642–649

32. Ravinet Trillou C, Delgorge C, Menet C, Arnone M, Soubrié P. CB1 cannabinoid receptor knockout in mice leads to leanness, resistance to diet-induced obesity and enhanced leptin sensitivity. *Int J Obes* (Lond) 2004;28:640–648

33. Migrenne S, Lacombe A, Lefèvre A-L, et al. Adiponectin is required to mediate rimonabant-induced improvement of insulin sensitivity but not body weight loss in diet-induced obese mice. *Am J Physiol Regul Integr Comp Physiol* 2009;296:R929–R935

34. Sowers JR. Endocrine functions of adipose tissue: focus on adiponectin. *Clin Cornerstone* 2008;9:32–38

35. Després J-P, Golay A, Sjöström L. Effects of rimonabant on metabolic risk factors in overweight patients with dyslipidemia. *N Engl J Med* 2005;353:2121–2134

36. Wierzbicki A, Pendleton S, McMahon Z, et al. Rimonabant improves cholesterol, insulin resistance and markers of non-alcoholic fatty liver in morbidly obese patients: a retrospective cohort study. *Int J Clin Pract* 2011;65:713–715

37. Viveros MP, Llorente R, Moreno E, Marco EM. Behavioural and neuroendocrine effects of cannabinoids in critical developmental periods. *Behav Pharmacol* 2005;16:353–362

38. Schlaepfer TE, Lancaster E, Heidbreder R, Strain EC, Kosel M, Fisch HU, Pearlson GD. Decreased frontal white-matter volume in chronic substance abuse. *Int J Neuropsychopharmacol* 2006;9:147–153

39. Linszen D, van Amelsvoort T. Cannabis and psychosis: an update on course and biological plausible mechanisms. *Curr Opin Psychiatry* 2007;20:116–120

40. Becker MP, Collins PF, Luciana M. Neurocognition in college-aged daily marijuana users. *J Clin Exp Neuropsychol* 2014;36:379–398

41. Leslie RD, Pyke DA, Stubbs WA. Sensitivity to enkephalin as a cause of non-insulin dependent diabetes. *Lancet* 1979;1:341–343

42. Giugliano D. Morphine, opioid peptides, and pancreatic islet function. *Diabetes Care* 1984;7:92–98

43. Giugliano D, Torella R, Lefèbvre PJ, D'Onofrio F. Opioid peptides and metabolic regulation. *Diabetologia* 1988;31:3–15

44. Giugliano D, Ceriello A, di Pinto P, Saccomanno F, Gentile S, Cappiapuoti F. Impaired insulin secretion in human diabetes mellitus. The effect of naloxone-induced opiate receptor blockade. *Diabetes* 1982;31:367–370

45. Passariello N, Giugliano D, Ceriello A, Chiariello A, Sgambato S, D'Onofrio F. Impaired insulin response to glucose but not to arginine in heroin addicts. *J Endocrinol Invest* 1986;9:353–357

46. Mason JS, Heber D. Endogenous opiates modulate insulin secretion in flushing noninsulin-dependent diabetics. *J Clin Endocrinol Metab* 1982;54:693–697

47. Evans AA, Tunnicliffe G, Knights P, Bailey CJ, Smith ME. Delta opioid receptors mediate glucose uptake in skeletal muscles of lean and obese-diabetic (ob/ob) mice. *Metabolism* 2001;50:1402–1408

48. Sadava D, Alonso D, Hong H, Pettit-Barrett DP. Effect of methadone addiction on glucose metabolism in rats. *Gen Pharmacol* 1997;28:27–29

49. Vuong C, Van Uum SH, O'Dell LE, Lutfy K, Friedman TC. The effects of opioids and opioid analogs on animal and human endocrine systems. *Endocr Rev* 2010;31:98–132

50. Levine AS, Morley JE, Gosnell BA, Billington CJ, Bartness TJ. Opioids and consummatory behavior. *Brain Res Bull* 1985;14:663–672

51. Levine AS, Billington CJ. Opioids. Are they regulators of feeding? *Ann NY Acad Sci* 1989;575:209–219

52. Baile CA, McLaughlin CL, Della-Fera MA. Role of cholecystokinin and opioid peptides in control of food intake. *Physiol Rev* 1986;66:172–234

53. Atkinson RL, Berke LK, Drake CR, Bibbs ML, Williams FL, Kaiser DL. Effects of long-term therapy with naltrexone on body weight in obesity. *Clin Pharmacol Ther* 1985;38:419–422

54. Yanovski SZ, Yanovski JA. Naltrexone extended-release plus bupropion extended-release for treatment of obesity. *JAMA* 2015; 313:1213–1214

55. Ceriello A, Giugliano D, Dello Russo P, Sgambato S, D'Onofrio F. Increased glycosylated haemoglobin A1 in opiate addicts: evidence for a hyperglycaemic effect of morphine. *Diabetologia* 1982;22:379

56. Passariello N, Giugliano D, Quatraro A, Consoli G, Sgambato S, Torella R, D'Onofrio F. Glucose tolerance and hormonal responses in heroin addicts. A possible role for endogenous opiates in the pathogenesis of non-insulin-dependent diabetes. *Metabolism* 1983;32:1163–1165

57. Mugunthan N, Davoren P. Danger of hypoglycemia due to acute tramadol poisoning. *Endocr Pract* 2012;18:e151–e152

58. Fournier JP, Azoulay L, Yin H, Montastruc JL, Suissa S. Tramadol use and the risk of hospitalization for hypoglycemia in patients with noncancer pain. *JAMA Intern Med* 2015;175:186–193

59. Manchikanti L, Helm S II, Fellows B, et al. Opioid epidemic in the United States. *Pain Physician* 2012;15(Suppl.):ES9–ES38

60. Cheng JT, Liu IM, Chi TC, Tzeng TF, Lu FH, Chang CJ. Plasma glucose-lowering effect of tramadol in streptozotocin-induced diabetic rats. *Diabetes* 2001;50:2815–2821

61. Choi SB, Jang JS, Park S. Tramadol enhances hepatic insulin sensitivity via enhancing insulin signaling cascade in the cerebral cortex and hypothalamus of 90% pancreatectomized rats. *Brain Res Bull* 2005;67:77–86

62. Nelson LS, Juurlink DN. Tramadol and hypoglycemia: one more thing to worry about. *JAMA Intern Med* 2015;175:194–195

63. Warner EA, Greene GS, Buchsbaum MS, Cooper DS, Robinson BE. Diabetic ketoacidosis associated with cocaine use. *Arch Intern Med* 1998;158:1799–1802

64. Abraham MR, Khardori R. Hyperglycemic hyperosmolar nonketotic syndrome as initial presentation of type 2 diabetes in a young cocaine abuser. *Diabetes Care* 1999;22:1380–1381

65. Nyenwe EA, Loganathan RS, Blum S, et al. Active use of cocaine: an independent risk factor for recurrent diabetic ketoacidosis in a city hospital. *Endocr Pract* 2007;13:22–29

66. Chiueh CC, Kopin IJ. Centrally mediated release by cocaine of endogenous epinephrine and norepinephrine from the sympathoad renal medullary system of unanesthetized rats. *J Pharmacol Exp Ther* 1978;205:148–154

67. Teoh SK, Sarnyai Z, Mendelson JH, Mello NK, Springer SA, Sholar JW, Walper M, Heesch CM, Negus BH, Keffer JH, Snyder RW, Risser RC, Eichhorn EJ. Effects of cocaine on cortisol secretion in humans. *Am J Med Sci* 1995;310:61–64

68. Heesch C, Negus B, Keffer J, Snyder R, Risser R, Eichhorn E. Effects of cocaine on cortisol secretion in humans. *Am J Med Sci* 1995;310:61–64

69. Cryer PE. Physiology and pathophysiology of the human sympathoadrenal neuroendocrine system. *N Engl J Med* 1980;303:436–444

70. Nurnberger JI Jr, Simmons-Alling S, Kessler L, et al. Separate mechanisms for behavioral, cardiovascular, and hormonal responses to dextroamphetamine in man. *Psychopharmacology* 1984;84:200–204

71. Nonogaki K. New insights into sympathetic regulation of glucose and fat metabolism. *Diabetologia* 2000;43:533–549

72. Branis NM, Wittlin SD. Amphetamine-like analogues in diabetes: speeding towards ketogenesis. *Case Rep Endocrinol* 2015;2015:917869. doi: 10.1155/2015/917869. Epub 2015 Apr 19

73. Isidro ML, Jorge S. Recreational drug abuse in patients hospitalized for diabetic ketosis or diabetic ketoacidosis. *Acta Diabetol* 2013;50:183–187

74. Garvey WT. Phentermine and topiramate extended-release: a new treatment for obesity and its role in a complications-centric approach to obesity medical management. *Expert Opinion on Drug Safety* 2013;12:741–756

11

Miscellaneous Agents

NONSTEROIDAL ANTI-INFLAMMATORY DRUGS, GLUCOSAMINE, AND ACETAMINOPHEN

Hyperglycemia is rarely reported in patients receiving nonsteroidal anti-inflammatory drugs (NSAIDs);[1] the mechanism for this is obscure, and a causal relationship is doubtful. Medically prescribed as well as over-the-counter products containing glucosamine sulfate are being used increasingly for the treatment or palliation of osteoarthritis. In animal studies, administration of glucosamine results in impaired secretion and action of insulin.[2] Increased substrate flux through the hexosamine pathway could be a mechanism for insulin resistance following exposure to glucosamine.[3] Studies in humans, however, have failed to show significant alterations in glucose tolerance, insulin sensitivity, or insulin action following treatment with oral glucosamine (500 mg tid) for 4 weeks.[4] In patients with established diabetes receiving antidiabetic medications, concurrent exposure to glucosamine did not alter glycemic control.[5] People with impaired glucose tolerance appear to be at increased risk for worsening dysglycemia following ingestion of glucosamine.[6] On the basis of human data, it is unlikely that the use of glucosamine in the recommended dosage would pose a significant risk for diabetes in people with normal glucose tolerance.

It would be advisable for people with risk factors for diabetes (Table 1.1) to undergo blood glucose screening before initiating glucosamine supplementation. If the screening test indicates prediabetes, lifestyle modification for diabetes risk reduction should be considered.

Ingestion of high doses of aspirin (4–6 g/day) or toxic overdose can cause hypoglycemia.[7,8] Salicylates are known to improve glucose tolerance via complex mechanisms, including enhanced insulin sensitivity, deceased gluconeogenesis, and decreased inflammatory cytokines.[9,10] These properties suggest that salicylates might decrease diabetes risk, although that conclusion awaits formal proof in human experimentation. The risk of hypoglycemia is minimal with lower doses of aspirin used for cardiovascular prophylaxis or routine pain control. Among obese patients with established type 2 diabetes (T2D), a randomized, placebo-controlled trial of salsalate (3.5 g/day) resulted in ~0.5% decrease in HbA$_{1c}$ after 6 months in the treated group compared with placebo.[11] In addition to improved glycemic control, other favorable metabolic effects of salsalate in patients with diabetes included increased adiponectin and decreased white blood cell triglyceride, and uric acid levels. Surprisingly, salsalate treatment did not improve endothelial dysfunction, and was associated with increased levels of low-density lipoprotein (LDL) cholesterol and urinary albumin excretion.[11,12] The mechanisms and clinical significance of the adverse lipid and renal effects need to be better understood before salsalate can be recommended for the management or prevention of diabetes.

Standard doses of acetaminophen, a widely used, over-the-counter analgesic and antipyretic, have not been associated directly with increased or decreased glucose production. Acetaminophen, however, has been reported to affect the accuracy of blood glucose readings from continuous glucose monitoring (CGM) devices. Glucose values reported by CGM could be falsely elevated in people taking acetaminophen. In a recent study, CGM readings were more than twofold higher than finger-stick readings following ingestion of acetaminophen.[13] In that study, patients with diabetes wearing a CGM device performed finger-stick blood glucose measurements at 30 min and 1, 2, 4, 6, and 8 h after ingesting 1,000 mg of acetaminophen. Significant differences were noted between the CGM and finger-stick blood glucose meter readings throughout the 8-h period of study, with the greatest discordance occurring at 2 h.[13] The differences between CGM and finger-stick blood glucose meter readings were greater in women than men, but they were not correlated with age, BMI, HbA_{1c} levels, or prevailing insulin regimen.[13]

The mechanism of the acetaminophen interference with CGM readings is not fully understood. It has been suggested that oxidation of the phenolic moiety in acetaminophen at the sensing electrode of certain glucose sensors (e.g., those measuring hydrogen peroxide) can produce a nonglycemic electrochemical signal that could interfere with glucose readings.[14,15] Manufacturers of CGM devices have been aware of the phenomenon and have issued a warning in the user guides about acetaminophen interference with the devices. Clinicians who order CGM for the purpose of understanding glycemic profiles in selected patients should ask such patients about acetaminophen use when interpreting the CGM output. Whenever feasible, patients should be advised to withhold acetaminophen 1–2 days before initiation of CGM. That interval should be sufficient to avoid significant interference, as the half-life of acetaminophen is ~3 h and complete urinary excretion of a 10 mg/kg oral dose occurs within 30 h.[16] It bears emphasizing that treatment decisions (especially, insulin dose adjustments) must be based on accurate information on ambient glycemic profile. Indeed, the current U.S. Food and Drug Administration (FDA) recommendation is that insulin dose calculations should be based on finger-stick blood glucose monitor results.

THYROID HORMONE

Thyroid hormone is one of the most widely prescribed medications in the general population, accounting for >70 million prescriptions each year in the U.S.[17] There is little evidence that physiological doses of thyroid hormone replacement significantly alter glucose regulation. In hyperthyroid patients, serum total T3 levels have been reported to correlate with glycosylated hemoglobin levels.[18] The mechanism for hyperthyroidism-associated dysglycemia probably involves increased glucose-6-phosphatase activity, increased hepatic glucose production, and possible alterations in insulin action and secretion.[19–21] The clinical import of the association between hyperthyroidism and glucose intolerance (even in people with established diabetes) is moot, as the overt hyperthyroidism is unlikely to be left untreated. Rare episodes of diabetic ketoacidosis have been reported in patients with untreated thyrotoxicosis, sometimes in the setting of interferon therapy for hepatitis C.[22–24] Nondiabetic ketoacidosis also has been reported as a complication of untreated severe hyperthyroidism.[25] Thyroid hormone potentiates the lipolytic actions of catecholamines in adipocytes and stimulates β-oxidation of fatty acids in hepatocytes.[26,27] Exaggeration of these processes in the setting of severe hyperthyroidism can create a ketogenic milieu.[28] In general, no special precautions or concerns regarding dysglycemia are called for in the routine treatment of hypothyroidism with standard thyroid hormone replacement in people with or without a history of diabetes.

PHENYTOIN AND ANTICONVULSANTS

Phenytoin is indicated for the control of generalized tonic-clonic, complex partial seizures, and treatment of status epilepticus. It is also widely prescribed for prophylaxis and treatment of seizures following head trauma or neurosurgery. Phenytoin has a narrow safety margin, and surveillance of drug levels is required during its use. Toxic doses of phenytoin have been associated with hyperglycemia, probably mediated by impaired insulin secretion.[29] In healthy young male volunteers, an intravenous (IV) loading dose of 15 mg/kg phenytoin resulted in acute increases in serum glucose and insulin levels, and a trend toward increased glucagon.[30]

It is unclear how these acute changes relate to glucoregulatory function during chronic oral treatment with phenytoin. Theoretically, the acute changes could worsen the hyperglycemia associated with seizures.[31] Although plasma levels of phenytoin within the therapeutic range (10–20 μ/ml) do not alter glucoregulation,[32] exacerbation of hyperglycemia and diabetic ketoacidosis have been reported in association with oral phenytoin treatment in patients with diabetes and seizure disorders.[33] Because the diabetic state can alter the pharmacokinetics of phenytoin,[34] careful monitoring of drug levels and glycemic control is warranted in patients with diabetes.

In addition to their use in patients with seizure disorders, anticonvulsants are used widely for the palliation of neuropathic pain in diabetes. In that setting, these agents are administered to patients with diabetes who are receiving concurrent antidiabetes medications, and disruption in glycemic control has not been a clinical problem. Weight gain is a common adverse effect of some anticonvulsant drugs, including carbamazepine, valproate, and gabapentin.[35] Significant weight gain, on a background of genetic risk, can increase the risk of diabetes. There have been no reports, however, of treatment-emergent diabetes following routine treatment with anticonvulsants.

GROWTH HORMONE

Patients with acromegaly have an increased risk of developing T2D, because of the metabolic effects of growth hormone (GH). During the past few decades, clinical indications for treatment with recombinant human GH have expanded to include short stature from GH deficiency in childhood, HIV cachexia, and GH deficiency in older adults, among others. The expanded uses of GH have been associated with reports of treatment-emergent diabetes and dysglycemia in both pediatric and elderly populations.[36,37] GH dose-dependently stimulates lipolysis, increases free fatty acids, induces insulin resistance, and decreases glucose oxidation.[38,39] The glucoregulatory system is exquisitely sensitive to the antagonistic effects of GH on insulin action.[40] For example, the physiological early morning increases in plasma GH levels do decrease insulin sensitivity in healthy subjects[38,41] and also explain the dawn phenomenon of morning hyperglycemia in patients with diabetes.[42]

Because of its appeal in popular culture (antiaging movement), possible surreptitious use, and imprecisions in the current methods for dosing GH, the scope of GH-induced hyperglycemia is likely to increase in future. The metabolic effects of GH predict that people with prediabetes or other risk factors for diabetes (Table 1.1) would be particularly at risk for hyperglycemia following exposure to pharmacological doses of GH. It is prudent, therefore, to obtain information on diabetes risk factors and to establish baseline fasting plasma glucose levels before initiating GH therapy. People with diabetes or prediabetes should be monitored closely and managed appropriately for any glycemic escalation.

TOTAL PARENTERAL NUTRITION AND INPATIENT HYPERGLYCEMIA

Although not strictly a drug, total parenteral nutrition (TPN) is given almost routinely to patients with critical illness and other inpatients undergoing prolonged restriction of oral intake. Hyperglycemia is a frequent finding in patients receiving TPN and has been associated with adverse outcomes in retrospective studies.[43,44] In one study, 457 patients receiving TPN were stratified by mean plasma glucose levels into quartiles: quartile 1 (<114 mg/dL), quartile 2 (114 to 137 mg/dL), quartile 3 (137 to 180 mg/dL), and quartile 4 (>180 mg/dL).[44] Logistic regression analysis showed that the odds ratio of death increased progressively by two- to fivefold from quartile 2 to quartile 4, compared with quartile 1. Each 10–mg/dL increase in mean blood glucose level was associated with increased risks for sepsis, cardiac complications, and renal failure.[44] A similar pattern of complications, and an even greater odds ratio of death (tenfold for quartile 4 compared with quartile 1), was reported by Cheung et al.[43] 5 in their retrospective study of 111 critically ill patients receiving TPN who developed hyperglycemia.

Mechanisms

The mechanisms underlying TPN-induced hyperglycemia are probably similar to the general mechanisms proposed for hyperglycemia in critically ill patients (stress of illness, glucocorticoids and other medications, prolonged immobilization, exacerbation of preexisting dysglycemia, etc.).[45] Furthermore, IV delivery of nutrients via TPN bypasses the intestinal incretin-secreting cells. Incretins, released by gut cells in response to oral food intake, augment insulin secretion and suppress glucagon. Without the help of incretins, IV nutrients fail to elicit adequate insulin secretion or glucagon suppression, leading to exaggerated postprandial hyperglycemia. In addition, the TPN solution often contains varying concentrations of dextrose that can contribute directly to hyperglycemia. The further mechanisms linking TPN-induced hyperglycemia to increased mortality and morbidity are not known precisely, although inflammatory cytokines and oxidative stress may play a role.[46]

Clearly, observational studies cannot separate the effects of underlying illness from those of TPN-induced hyperglycemia. Therefore, a prospective, randomized, controlled study (with an intervention arm that achieves normoglycemia in TPN-treated patients) is needed to confirm causal associations between hyperglycemia and increased mortality and morbidity.

Approach to Management and Risk Reduction

Glycemic Targets. No randomized controlled studies have been conducted specifically to determine optimal glycemic targets for patients receiving TPN. In the absence of such data, an empirical approach, based on extrapolations from studies on inpatient hyperglycemia, is a viable option. A reasonable and evidence-based target for surgical patients in critical care units appears to be a blood glucose level of 80–110 mg/dL, which was demonstrated by van den Berghe et al.[47-49] to decrease mortality. The NICE-SUGAR (Normoglycemia in Intensive Care Evaluation-Survival Using Glucose Algorithm Regulation) study results, however, are in sharp discord with the dramatic benefits observed in the reports by van den Berghe et al..[47-50] On the basis of the pooled data in a meta-analysis of 26 trials (including NICE-SUGAR) with a total of 13,567 hospitalized patients, it was concluded that there was no mortality benefit, but a sixfold increased risk of hypoglycemia, from intensive glycemic control (compared with conventional therapy).[51] The pooled data confirmed that patients in surgical intensive care units (ICUs) benefited significantly from intensive insulin therapy with a mortality risk reduction of 47% (consistent with van den Berghe et al.[47]), whereas there was no significant benefit for patients in medical ICUs.[51] Thus, intensive insulin therapy increased the risk of hypoglycemia without benefit on mortality in critically ill patients, except in the subgroup of those admitted to the surgical ICU.[51-54] In the NICE-SUGAR study, patients assigned to the conventional treatment group had a mean blood glucose level of 144 mg/dL and had better outcomes than the intensively treated group. Thus, target blood glucose values of ~140 mg/dL would appear to be reasonable for inpatients. It is no longer considered necessary or safe to pursue aggressive control of blood glucose to levels of <110 mg/dL in the hospitalized patient. The joint consensus statement from American Association of Clinical Endocrinologists (AACE) and the American Diabetes Association (ADA) recommends less stringent glycemic targets for patients in intensive care units as well as those admitted to general medical and surgical wards.[55] For critically ill patients in the ICU setting, the current recommendation is to initiate insulin infusion to control hyperglycemia in patients whose blood glucose levels are >180 mg/dL and to maintain blood glucose level between 140 mg/dL and 180 mg/dL.[55,56] Those are reasonable glycemic targets for patients with TPN-associated hyperglycemia as well, pending randomized controlled trials to address the specific question. The same glycemic targets have been recommended for noncritically ill hospitalized patients.[57-59]

Choice of Antihyperglycemic Agent. In most cases, the underlying indications for suspension of oral intake and institution of TPN would preclude the use of oral hypoglycemic agents for managing TPN-induced hyperglycemia. Similarly, the prolonged action of subcutaneous insulin makes that a risky option in a patient whose sole caloric intake depends on TPN. Any technical problems that lead to interruption of TPN (e.g., loss of venous access) would expose such a patient to the risk of severe hypoglycemia from the continued absorption of insulin from subcutaneous sites. For these reasons, IV insulin infusion is the regimen of choice for controlling TPN-induced hyperglycemia, whenever adequate skilled nursing staff is available to monitor the patient. Regular, short-acting insulin should be used for IV infusion, because there is no advantage to using the more expensive rapid-acting analogs, which are designed for faster absorption from subcutaneous sites. The insulin can be administered via a separate infusion or mixed with the TPN solution. The separate infusion allows greater flexibility but requires closer monitoring by skilled nurses.[60]

If IV insulin infusion cannot be administered safely due to lack of adequate nursing coverage, multiple injections of subcutaneous insulin may be used to maintain desirable blood glucose targets. Because of their shorter duration of action, subcutaneous administration of rapid-acting insulin analogs may pose a lower risk of prolonged hypoglycemia in the event of TPN interruption, compared with regular insulin. Bedside blood glucose should be monitored frequently (Q 1--2 h during IV insulin infusion and Q 3–4 h for subcutaneous regimen). A written protocol (algorithm) for adjustment of insulin infusion rates in relation to ambient glucose levels should be created to direct nursing staff in the safe management of hyperglycemia. Numerous algorithms and guidelines for insulin infusion have been published[56] and many hospitals have developed their own local guidelines; however, the best algorithm is one that is flexible, individualized, and tailored to the changing needs and condition of the patients.

REFERENCES

1. Tkach JR. Indomethacin-induced hyperglycemia in psoriatic arthritis. *J Am Acad Dermatol* 1982;7:802–803
2. Giaccari A, Morviducci L, Zoretta D, et al. In vivo effects of glucosamine on insulin secretion and insulin sensitivity in rat: possible relevance to the maladaptive responses to chronic hyperglycemia. *Diabetologia* 1995;38:518–524
3. Monauni T, Zenti MG, Cretti A, et al. Effects of glucosamine infusion on insulin secretion and insulin action in humans. *Diabetes* 2000;49:926–935
4. Yu JG, Boies SM, Olefsky JM. The effect of oral glucosamine sulfate on insulin sensitivity in human subjects. *Diabetes Care* 2003;26:1941–1942
5. Scroggie DA, Albright A, Harris MD. The effect of glucosamine-chondroitin supplementation on glycosylated hemoglobin levels in patients with type

2 diabetes mellitus. A placebo-controlled, double-blinded, randomized clinical trial. *Arch Intern Med* 2003;163:1587–1590

6. Biggee BA, Blinn CM, Nuite M, Silbert JE, McAlindon TE. Effects of oral glucosamine sulphate on serum glucose and insulin during an oral glucose tolerance test of subjects with osteoarthritis. *Ann Rheum Dis* 2007;66:260–262

7. Cotton EK, Fahlberg YI. Hypoglycemia with salicylate poisoning. *Am J Dis Child* 1964;108:171–173

8. Gilgore SG. The influence of salicylate on hyperglycemia. *Diabetes* 1960; 9:392–393

9. Netea MG, Tack CJ, Netten PM, Lutterman JA, Van der Meer JW. The effect of salicylates on insulin sensitivity. *J Clin Invest* 2001;108:1723–1724

10. Hundal RS, Petersen KF, Mayerson AB, et al. Mechanism by which high-dose aspirin improves glucose metabolism in type 2 diabetes. *J Clin Invest* 2002;109:1321–1326

11. Goldfine AB, Fonseca V, Jablonski KA, Pyle L, Staten MA, Shoelson SE; TINSAL-T2D (Targeting Inflammation Using Salsalate in Type 2 Diabetes) Study Team. The effects of salsalate on glycemic control in patients with type 2 diabetes: a randomized trial. *Ann Intern Med* 2010;152:346–357

12. Goldfine AB, Buck JS, Desouza C, Fonseca V, Chen YD, Shoelson SE, Jablonski KA, Creager MA; TINSAL-FMD Ancillary Study Team. Targeting inflammation using salsalate in patients with type 2 diabetes: effects on flow-mediated dilation (TINSAL-FMD). *Diabetes Care* 2013;36:4132–4139

13. Maahs DM, DeSalvo D, Pyle L, et al. Effect of acetaminophen on CGM glucose in an outpatient setting. *Diabetes Care* 2015;38:e158–159

14. Zhang Y, Hu Y, Wilson GS, Moatti-Sirat D, Poitout V, Reach G. Elimination of the acetaminophen interference in an implantable glucose sensor. *Anal Chem* 1994;66:1183–1188

15. Moatti-Sirat D, Poitout V, Thom´e V, et al. Reduction of acetaminophen interference in glucose sensors by a composite Nafion membrane: demonstration in rats and man. *Diabetologia* 1994;37:610–616

16. Miller RP, Roberts RJ, Fischer LJ. Acetaminophen elimination kinetics in neonates, children, and adults. *Clin Pharmacol Ther* 1976;19:284–294

17. DeNoon DJ. The 10 most widely prescribed drugs. Available from http://www.webmd.com/news/20110420/the-10-most-prescribed-drugs. Accessed 3 July 2015

18. Saito T, Sato T, Yamamoto M, et al. Hemoglobin A1 levels in hyperthyroidism. *Endocrinol Jpn* 1982;29:137–140

19. Taylor R, McCulloch AJ, Zeuzem S, Gray P, Clark F, Alberti KG. Insulin secretion, adipocyte insulin binding and insulin sensitivity in thyrotoxicosis. *Acta Endocrinol* (Copenh) 1985;109:96–103

20. Cavallo-Perin P, Bruno A, Bozzo C, Boine L, Estivi P, Martina V, et al. Insulin binding to monocytes and in vivo peripheral insulin sensitivity are normal in Graves' disease. *J Endocrinol Invest* 1988;11:795–800

21. Karlander SG, Khan A, Wajngot A, Torring O, Vranic M, Efendic S. Glucose turnover in hyperthyroid patients with normal glucose tolerance. *J Clin Endocrinol Metab* 1989;68:780–786

22. Yeo KF, Yang YS, Chen KS, Peng CH, Huang CN. Simultaneous presentation of thyrotoxicosis and diabetic ketoacidosis resulted in sudden cardiac arrest. *Endocr J* 2007;54:991–993

23. Soultati AS, Dourakis SP, Alexopoulou A, Deutsch M, Archimandritis AJ. Simultaneous development of diabetic ketoacidosis and Hashitoxicosis in a patient treated with pegylated interferon-alpha for chronic hepatitis C. *World J Gastroenterol* 2007;13:1292–1294

24. Hayashi M, Kataoka Y, Tachikawa K, Koguchi H, Tanaka H. Dual onset of type 1 diabetes mellitus and Graves' disease during treatment with pegylated interferon alpha-2b and ribavirin for chronic hepatitis C. *Diabetes Res Clin Pract* 2009;86:e19–21

25. Wood ET, Kinlaw WB. Nondiabetic ketoacidosis caused by severe hyperthyroidism. *Thyroid* 2004;14:628–630

26. Hellstrom L, Wahrenberg H, Reynisdottir S, Arner P. Catecholamine-induced adipocyte lipolysis in human hyperthyroidism. *J Clin Endocrinol Metab* 1997;82:159–166

27. Müller M, Acheson K, Jequier E, Burger A. Thyroid hormone action on lipid metabolism in humans: A role for endogenous insulin. *Metabolism* 1990;39:480–485

28. Keller U, Lustenberger M, Müller-Brand J, Gerber P, Stauffacher W. Human ketone body production and utilization studies using tracer techniques: Regulation by free fatty acids, insulin, catecholamines, and thyroid hormones. *Diabetes Metab Rev* 1989;5:285–298

29. Fariss BL, Lutcher CL. Diphenylhydantoin-induced hyperglycemia and impaired insulin release. Effect of dosage. *Diabetes* 1971;20:177–181

30. Banner W Jr, Johnson DG, Walson PD, Jung D. Effects of single large doses of phenytoin on glucose homeostasis—a preliminary report. *J Clin Pharmacol* 1982;22:79–81

31. Huang CW, Tsai JJ, Ou HY, Wang ST, Cheng JT, Wu SN, Huang CC. Diabetic hyperglycemia is associated with the severity of epileptic seizures in adults. *Epilepsy Res* 2008;79:71–77

32. Callaghan N, Feely M, O'Callaghan M, Duggan B, McGarry J, Cramer B, et al. The effects of toxic and non-toxic serum phenytoin levels on carbohydrate tolerance and insulin levels. *Acta Neurol Scand* 1977;56:563–571

33. Carter BL, Small RE, Mandel MD, Starkman MT. Phenytoin-induced hyperglycemia. *Am J Hosp Pharm* 1981;38:1508–1512

34. Adithan C, Srinivas B, Indhiresan J, et al. Influence of type I and type II diabetes mellitus on phenytoin steady-state levels. *Int J Clin Pharmacol Ther Toxicol* 1991;29:310–313

35. Jallon P, Picard F. Bodyweight gain and anticonvulsants: a comparative review. *Drug Saf* 2001;24:969–978

36. Czernichow P. Growth hormone administration and carbohydrate metabolism. *Horm Res* 1993;39:102–103

37. Bramnert M, Segerlantz M, Laurila E, Daugaard JR, Manhem P, Groop L. Growth hormone replacement therapy induces insulin resistance by activating the glucose-fatty acid cycle. *J Clin Endocrinol Metab* 2003;88:1455–1463

38. Bratusch-Marrain PR, Smith D, DeFronzo RA. The effect of growth hormone on glucose metabolism and insulin secretion in man. *J Clin Endocrinol Metab* 1982;55:973–982

39. Salgin B, Marcovecchio ML, Williams RM, et al. Effects of growth hormone and free fatty acids on insulin sensitivity in patients with type 1 diabetes. *J Clin Endocrinol Metab* 2009; 94:3297–3305

40. Holly JMP, Amiel SA, Sandhu RR, Rees LH, Wass JAH. The role of growth hormone in diabetes mellitus. *J Endocrinol* 1988;118:353–364

41. Rizza RA, Mandarino LJ, Gerich JE. Effects of growth hormone on insulin action in man. Mechanisms of insulin resistance, impaired suppression of glucose production, and impaired stimulation of glucose utilization. *Diabetes* 1982;31:663–669

42. Møller N, Jørgensen JO. Effects of growth hormone on glucose, lipid, and protein metabolism in human subjects. *Endocr Rev* 2009;30:152–177

43. Cheung NW, Napier B, Zaccaria C, Fletcher JP. Hyperglycemia is associated with adverse outcomes in patients receiving total parenteral nutrition. *Diabetes Care* 2005;28:2367–2371

44. Lin LY, Lin HC, Lee PC, Ma WY, Lin HD. Hyperglycemia correlates with outcomes in patients receiving total parenteral nutrition. *Am J Med Sci* 2007;333:261–265

45. Dagogo-Jack S, Alberti KGMM. Diabetes mellitus in surgical patients. *Diabetes Spect* 2002;15:44–48

46. Esposito K, Nappo F, Marfella R, et al. Inflammatory cytokine concentrations are acutely increased by hyperglycemia in humans: role of oxidative stress. *Circulation* 2002;106:2067–2072

47. van den Berghe G, Wouters P, Weekers F, Verwaest C, Bruyninckx F, Schetz M, Vlasselaers D, Ferdinande P, Lauwers P, Bouillon R. Intensive insulin therapy in the critically ill patients. *N Engl J Med* 2001;345:1359–1367

48. van den Berghe G, Wouters PJ, Bouillon R, Weekers F, Verwaest C, Schetz M, Vlasselaers D, Ferdinande P, Lauwers P. Outcome benefit of intensive insulin therapy in the critically ill: insulin dose versus glycemic control. *Crit Care Med* 2003;31:359–366

49. van den Berghe G, Wilmer A, Hermans G, Meersseman W, Wouters PJ, Milants I, Van Wijngaerden E, Bobbaers H, Bouillon R: Intensive insulin therapy in the medical ICU. *N Engl J Med* 2006;354:449–461

50. NICE-SUGAR Study Investigators, Finfer S, Chittock DR, et al. Intensive versus conventional glucose control in critically ill patients. *N Engl J Med* 2009;360:1283–1297

51. Griesdale DE, de Souza RJ, van Dam RM, et al. Intensive insulin therapy and mortality among critically ill patients: a meta-analysis including NICE-SUGAR study data. *CMAJ* 2009;180:821–827

52. Krinsley JS, Grover A. Severe hypoglycemia in critically ill patients: risk factors and outcomes. *Crit Care Med* 2007;35:2262–2267

52. Wiener RS, Wiener DC, Larson RJ. Benefits and risks of tight glucose control in critically ill adults: a meta-analysis. *JAMA* 2008;300:933–944

54. Brunkhorst FM, Engel C, Bloos F, et al. Intensive insulin therapy and pentastarch resuscitation in severe sepsis. *N Engl J Med* 2008;358:125–139

55. Moghissi ES, Korytkowski MT, DiNardo M, et al. American Association of Clinical Endocrinologists and American Diabetes Association consensus statement on inpatient glycemic control. *Diabetes Care* 2009;32:1119–1131

56. Jacobi J, Bircher N, Krinsley J, et al. Guidelines for the use of an insulin infusion for the management of hyperglycemia in critically ill patients. *Crit Care Med* 2012;40:3251–3276

57. Umpierrez GE, Hellman R, Korytkowski MT, Kosiborod M, Maynard GA, Montori VM, Seley JJ, Van den Berghe G. Management of hyperglycemia in hospitalized patients in non-critical care setting: an Endocrine Society clinical practice guideline. *J Clin Endocrinol Metab* 2012;97:16–38

58. Murad MH, Coburn JA, Coto-Yglesias F, Dzyubak S, Hazem A, Lane MA, Prokop LJ, Montori VM. Glycemic control in non-critically ill hospitalized patients: a systematic review and meta-analysis. *J Clin Endocrinol Metab* 2012;97:49–58

59. American Diabetes Association. Diabetes care in the hospital, nursing home, and skilled nursing facility. *Diabetes Care* 2015;38(Suppl. 1):S80–S85

60. Knapke CM, Owens JP, Mirtallo JM. Management of glucose abnormalities in patients receiving total parenteral nutrition. *Clin Pharm* 1989;8:136–144

12

General Approach to
Risk Reduction

The first step toward reduction of the risk of iatrogenic hyperglycemia is a thoughtful evaluation of the indications for any prescription, which should be based on compelling evidence. Whenever feasible, medications of proven efficacy on the primary condition that exhibit a low risk for dysglycemia should be given preference, particularly in high-risk individuals. One example is the treatment of hypertension, for which a drug selection policy that favors angiotensin-converting enzyme (ACE) inhibitors, angiotensin receptor blockers (ARBs), or calcium-channel blocker CCBs over thiazides and β-blockers in high-risk subjects with prediabetes can be defended.[1]

In cases in which the use of a drug with an adverse glucose profile is unavoidable, prescription of the lowest effective dose, for the minimum duration, required to control the primary disorder is a reasonable approach to diabetes risk reduction. This concept is most applicable to the field of transplant immunosuppression and other steroid-requiring conditions. In general, minimization of dose and duration of drug treatment as a prudent strategy for diabetes risk reduction is applicable to antidepressants, nicotinic acid, β-adrenergic agonists, thiazides, β-blockers, and several other medications. In some instances, the potential adverse glycemic effects of a given drug class can be mitigated by choosing a compound with counterbalancing activities. For example, the use of a combined α- and β-adrenergic blocker (e.g., labetalol, carvedilol) often mitigates the adverse metabolic effects of a pure β-blocker. Furthermore, in the management of dyslipidemia in people with diabetes or prediabetes, the inclusion of agents that enhance glucose tolerance (e.g., fibrates and bile acid sequestrants) might help decrease the risk of glycemic exacerbation.

Whenever the evidence and the clinical condition permit, switching from a suspect drug to another equally efficacious agent that is known to have a better metabolic profile should be considered (Figure 12.1). If diabetes develops during treatment with a medication that cannot be withdrawn or substituted, a multimodality approach to glycemic control is advocated. That approach incorporates self–blood glucose monitoring, diabetes education, dietary counseling, physical activity, and selective use of antidiabetic medications. The mnemonic MEDEM (monitoring, education, diet, exercise, medication) can be used to recall the key modalities of diabetes management.

Figure 12.1—Drug Classes Associated with Glucose Abnormalities and General Approach to Risk Reduction

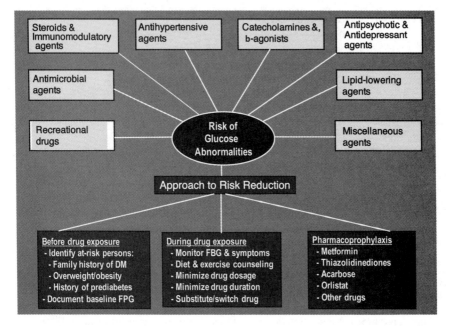

LIFESTYLE INTERVENTION FOR DIABETES PREVENTION

In people who require long-term treatment with a potentially diabetogenic drug, consideration should be given to lifestyle counseling for prevention of diabetes. The Diabetes Prevention Program (DPP) and other studies have shown that lifestyle modification in people with prediabetes can reduce the risk of progression to diabetes by ~60%.[2,3] Other studies have shown that lifestyle modification prevents weight gain in patients with schizophrenia treated with atypical antipsychotic drugs.[4,5] The DPP lifestyle intervention utilizes five key approaches that provide a general construct for counseling patients at risk for drug-induced hyperglycemia. The key approaches are enumerated for easier reference:

1. *Selection of people at risk.* The DPP utilized a risk factor–based approach to identify people who may benefit from intervention (Table 1.1). Specifically targeted were people with a family history of type 2 diabetes (T2D) who have a high BMI (>24 kg/m²) and fasting plasma glucose in the range of 96–125 mg/dL. The BMI cut-off was lowered to >22 kg/m² for Asians.
2. *Increased physical activity.* The DPP physical activity goal was 30 min of moderate-intensity aerobic activity (equivalent to brisk walking) for 5 days/week (total 150 min/week).

3. *Dietary intervention.* The participants were coached by dietitians to decrease fat calories to <30% and total calories by 500–700 kcal/day, by selectively reducing the intake of saturated fats and excessive carbohydrates.
4. *Weight-loss goal.* DPP participants were instructed and encouraged to have a weight-loss goal of at least 7%, and to maintain a healthy weight through the aforementioned lifestyle modifications.
5. *Self-monitoring.* The participants recorded their food intake and minutes spent performing physical activity each day. Self-monitoring behavior has been shown to predict long-term maintenance of weight loss and could well have been an important adjunct to the excellent results obtained in the DPP.

COMMUNITY RESOURCES

Several recognized diabetes prevention programs now are available in YMCAs and other community sites in the U.S. to which at-risk persons can be referred for counseling. Online diabetes prevention programs provided by Canary Health[6] and other agencies have also become available. It is noteworthy that more than 20 major insurers now cover these congressionally mandated diabetes prevention programs. Additional information regarding these programs can be accessed on the Centers for Disease Control and Prevention's (CDC's) website.[7] Prevent Diabetes STAT (Screen/Test/Act Today), a joint initiative sponsored by the CDC and the American Medical Association, also provides valuable information, action plans, and community resources for health care professionals and lay citizens.[8]

LIMITATIONS OF LIFESTYLE INTERVENTION

Most of the lifestyle intervention programs aimed at preventing diabetes have been designed as randomized controlled trials conducted predominantly at academic medical centers. These trials have involved frequent clinic visits, multidisciplinary teams (including physicians, nurses, dietitians, psychologists, exercise physiologists, and others), and substantial resources and support from funding agencies. Furthermore, the services were offered at no cost to the study subjects; indeed, participants in some of the studies received stipends for their participation. It remains to be shown whether the high rates of success achieved in the randomized controlled trials would be reproduced in routine clinical practice and in the community settings. Some community initiatives are currently underway to determine the feasibility of community programs for diabetes prevention,[9,10] with promising initial results.[11]

Even in the most successful of the randomized controlled trials, the risk reduction for incident diabetes following lifestyle intervention was ~60%.[2,3,12,13] These results raise the argument as to whether medications could be offered to high-risk people who are unable or unwilling to implement lifestyle changes, or in whom the latter have failed to halt glycemic progression. In fact, several of the landmark diabetes prevention trials also included pharmacological arms, and additional studies have specifically tested medications for diabetes prevention.

What follows is a summary of medications that have been studied for the prevention of T2D.

MEDICATIONS FOR DIABETES PREVENTION

Table 12.1 summarizes some randomized controlled studies that have tested the effects of lifestyle intervention and different medications on the progression from prediabetes to T2D. The list of medications that have been tested includes sulfonylureas, metformin, acarbose, orlistat, rosiglitazone, and pioglitazone. The DPP demonstrated that intervention with metformin decreased the development of diabetes in adults with impaired glucose tolerance by 31%.[2] Curiously, the diabetes prevention efficacy of metformin was observed only in younger, obese (BMI >35 kg/m^2) individuals; among older or leaner participants, the drug was no better than placebo in diabetes risk reduction.[2]

Table 12.1—Diabetes Prevention Studies Using Lifestyle Modification and Medications

Year	Study	Follow-up	Intervention	Outcome
1997	Da Qing	6 yr	Diet + exercise	Decrease, 51%
2001	DPS, Finland	3 yr	Diet + exercise	Decrease, 58%
2002	DPP	2.8 yr	Diet + ex vs. Met	Decrease, 58%
2002	STOP-NIDDM	3.3 yr	Acarbose + diet	Decrease, 25%
2004	XENdos	4 yr	Xenical + diet	Decrease, 37%
2006	DREAM	3 yr	Rosiglitazone	Decrease, 60%
2008	ACT NOW	2–4 yr	Pioglitazone	Decrease, 72%
2006	IDPP-1	3 yr	L/S ± Met	Decrease, 26–28% Met not additive to L/S
2009	IDPP-2	3 yr	L/S ± Pio	Pio not additive to L/S
2010	Navigator	5 yr	Nateglinide Valsartan	No effect Decrease, 14%
2010	CANOE	4 yr	Rosi + Met	Decrease, 69%

STOP-NIDDM (Study to Prevent Non-Insulin-Dependent Diabetes Mellitus) employed acarbose as the intervention drug, and demonstrated a 25% decrease in the rate of progression to diabetes, compared with placebo.[14] In the XENical in the Prevention of Diabetes in Obese Subjects (XENDOS) study, orlistat (a lipase inhibitor that is approved as a weightloss drug) in combination with lifestyle modification resulted in a 37% risk reduction in incident diabetes among subjects with impaired glucose tolerance, compared with lifestyle intervention alone.[15] Thiazolidinedione drugs were tested in several studies, including the Pioglitazone in the Prevention of Diabetes (PIPOD),[16] Diabetes Reduction Assessment with Ramipril and Rosiglitazone Medication (DREAM),[17] Actos Now for the Prevention of Diabetes (ACT NOW),[18] and Canadian Normoglycemia Outcomes Evaluation (CANOE),[19] which showed diabetes risk reduction rates of >50–75% compared with placebo.

In the NAVIGATOR trial, the use of valsartan for 5 years, along with lifestyle modification, led to a relative reduction of 14% in the incidence of diabetes among subjects with impaired glucose tolerance (IGT) [20a], but the effect of nateglinide was not better than placebo.[20b] The CANOE trial showed that low-dose combination therapy with metformin (500 mg twice daily) and rosiglitazone (2 mg daily) decreased incident T2D by 66% compared with placebo in IGT subjects. Of note, the low doses were well tolerated, with minimal effect on clinically relevant adverse events of the individual drugs.[19]

LIMITATIONS OF MEDICATIONS

The drugs that have been tested for diabetes prevention are associated with a range of adverse effects, the need for continuous therapy to maintain their effects, and consequent adherence barriers. In the studies that tested the effect of interruption of metformin and rosiglitazone therapy, a fairly rapid glycemic rebound was observed, which indicates that those medications did not fundamentally modify the underlying pathophysiology of prediabetes.[21,22] Equally disappointing is the observation in the Indian Diabetes Prevention Program (IDPP)-1 and IDPP-2 that low-dose metformin or pioglitazone, when tested in combination with lifestyle modification, did not result in additional reduction of diabetes risk, compared with the effects of lifestyle modification alone.[13,23] Moreover, the cumulative costs of long-term (probably lifelong) therapy with medications (even in cases in which generic versions are available) can be prohibitive, particularly for developing countries.[24]

Owing to the aforementioned concerns, the use of drugs for diabetes prevention cannot be recommended as a first-line approach in the general population. The latter conclusion is not to deny a societal expectation of safe, effective, and durable medications that could serve as alternatives or adjuncts to lifestyle intervention for diabetes prevention. The impetus for such an expectation is underscored by the poor human record of long-term adherence to dietary and exercise recommendations, as well as physiological adaptations that limit weight loss and induce regain in the weight-reduced state.[25] The ideal drug for diabetes prevention (Table 12.2) should be well tolerated and nontoxic, and its potency should match or surpass the efficacy of lifestyle modification.[24,26] Additionally, such a drug should be capable of repairing the pathophysiologic defects that underlie prediabetes, so that a durable effect that outlasts the period of medication can be expected. The latter attribute would permit withdrawal of the medication after a defined period of intervention, without the risk of prediabetes relapse.

Finally, the cost of such a drug must not be prohibitive, bearing in mind the large number of people with prediabetes (86 million in the U.S. and >400 million worldwide). To exert a lasting effect, a novel compound must significantly increase pancreatic β-cell mass, either by decreasing apoptosis, enhancing prolif-

Table 12.2—Desirable Characteristics of the Ideal Drug for Diabetes Prevention

■ Efficacy: should equal or exceed the efficacy of lifestyle intervention.

■ Mechanism(s): should repair the pathophysiologic defects that underlie prediabetes.

■ Glucoregulation: should normalize glucose metabolism.

■ Durability: effects should outlast the period of medication exposure.

■ Adiposity: should induce weight loss or be weight-neutral.

■ Safety: should have minimal toxicity and require no safety monitoring.

■ Tolerability: should be well-tolerated, without GI or other adverse effects.

■ Cost: should cost less than the least expensive drug for diabetes treatment.

Source: Modified from Edeoga and Dagogo-Jack.[26]

eration, inducing neogenesis, or trans-differentiating endoderm-derived cells into insulin-making cells.[24,27] Additional effects on amelioration of insulin resistance also would be desirable.

The discovery of pharmaceutical agents with the aforementioned properties could engender a novel approach to diabetes prevention that entails drug treatment for a defined period (say, 3–6 months), followed by drug withdrawal, without the risk of rebound in blood glucose levels. In other words, a vaccination model for diabetes prevention. Currently, none of the available drugs meets all the desirable criteria of the ideal diabetes prevention drug. It may be possible, however, to design a drug or a combination of drugs that can meet most of the desired criteria. A medication that improves insulin sensitivity through induction of significant weight loss, along with improving β-cell function (perhaps through cellular growth, regeneration, or antiapoptosis) could have a durable effect in reversing the prediabetes phenotype. The incretins, incretin analogs, incretin-mimetic drugs, and newer antiobesity medications offer some promising perspectives in this direction. Further evaluation of these agents and other potent compounds alone and in combination with lifestyle interventions is warranted.

CURRENT GUIDELINES FOR USE OF MEDICATIONS FOR DIABETES PREVENTION

The American Diabetes Association (ADA) consensus statement[28] recommends lifestyle modification with a weight-loss goal of 5–10% along with moderate physical activity of about 30 min daily for patients with impaired fasting glucose (IFG) or IGT. Although no drug has yet been approved by the U.S. Food and Drug Administration (FDA) for diabetes prevention, the ADA has suggested that treatment with metformin be considered as an adjunct to diet and exercise for the prevention of T2D in selected high-risk persons.[28,29] On the basis of the subgroup analysis of the efficacy of metformin in the DPP,[2] metformin was most effective in preventing diabetes in high-risk, obese (BMI >35 kg/m^2) subjects with prediabetes <60 years of age.[2] Additional selection criteria when considering metformin use in subjects with prediabetes include a family history of diabetes in first-degree relatives, prior gestational diabetes mellitus, hypertiglyceridemia, subnormal high-density lipoprotein cholesterol levels, hypertension, and HbA$_{1c}$ 5.7–6.4%.[28,29]

Even in people who harbor all or most of these risk factors, active lifestyle modification must be the initial intervention, with the addition of metformin considered for individuals who fail to make significant progress. Currently, there are no clear guidelines for determining the optimal timing of metformin therapy, but failure of lifestyle intervention can be determined fairly empirically. The DPP participants assigned to lifestyle intervention lost ~7% of their baseline body weight during the first 6 months. Thus, one practical rule of thumb might be a weight loss goal of 1% per month during the initial 3–6 months of lifestyle intervention. High-risk individuals who are unable to meet such a target may be considered for metformin. Guidelines on the management of prediabetes, issued by the Indian Health Services (IHS) and the Australian Diabetes Society/Australian Diabetes Educators Association, also emphasize lifestyle intervention, with judicious use of medications. The Australian guidelines recommend lifestyle intervention as first-line therapy for a minimum of 6 months before consideration of pharmacotherapy.[30] The IHS guidelines recommend that lifestyle interventions should be the primary focus for diabetes prevention and that either metformin or pioglitizone be considered if further glucose control is needed.[1] The IHS guidelines state that the decision to use medication for diabetes prevention must be made on an individual basis and with the patient's full understanding.[1]

Biochemically, an individual can be diagnosed with prediabetes on the basis of having an IFG alone, IGT alone (determined during oral glucose tolerance test), or both IFG and IGT. Individuals who have both IFG and IGT (double prediabetes) show more severe insulin resistance and impairment of β-cell function compared with people who have a single prediabetes marker.[28,31,32] It has been estimated that most individuals (~96%) with double prediabetes would qualify for metformin therapy, based on the ADA consensus criteria.[28,33] By contrast, only ~30% of people with IFG would meet the criteria for metformin treatment, using the same criteria. This means that a strategy for comprehensive risk stratification and preventive intervention should include oral glucose tolerance testing, to identify individuals with IFG who also harbor coexisting IGT and thus may be candidates for adjunctive metformin treatment.[28,33] Indeed, the ADA consensus statement stipulates that the presence of both IFG and IGT must be documented if metformin is to be used for diabetes prevention.[28]

DIABETES PHARMACOPROPHYLAXIS

The question often arises as to whether high-risk patients receiving chronic treatment with potentially diabetogenic agents (e.g., steroids) should receive prior or concurrent prophylactic therapy with medications to prevent diabetes. The concept is attractive and needs to be developed further. When is the best time for starting such prophylactic treatment—before or after initiation of the known diabetogenic therapy? How long before, or how long after, exposure to a diabetogenic drug should diabetes prophylaxis be started? Does the prophylactic treatment need to overlap completely with the duration of exposure to the diabetogenic therapy, or can a rationale for more precise timing be developed, based on pharmacokinetic and pharmacodynamics data? How often should blood glucose be monitored during such a regimen? And what else besides glucose should be tracked? Which medications would be appropriate to consider for diabetes prophylaxis? What is the threshold for selecting patients for diabetes prophylaxis?

Unfortunately, there is no specific, evidence-based information to provide answers for the numerous open questions. Clearly, randomized controlled studies are needed to demonstrate whether diabetes pharmacoprophylaxis is a rational strategy in high-risk people who are receiving treatment with potentially diabetogenic drugs. Obvious drug candidates for such randomized controlled trials would be metformin, thiazolidinediones, acarbose, and orlistat (all of which have pertinent preliminary data); metformin, in particular, has long-term efficacy and safety data from the DPP Outcomes Study.[34] The dipeptidyl peptidase-4 (DPP-4) inhibitors (e.g., sitagliptin, vildagliptin, saxagliptin, linagliptin, alogliptin), sodium glucose cotransporter 2 (SGLT2) inhibitors (e.g., canagliflozin, dapagliflozin, empagliflozin), and the dopamine agonist bromocriptine-QR also may be attractive trial candidates because of their low risk for iatrogenic hypoglycemia and interesting mechanisms of action.[35] Furthermore, randomized controlled trials of pharmacoprophylaxis with the glucagon-like peptide-1 (GLP-1) receptor agonists (e.g., exenatide, liraglutide, albiglutide, dulaglutide) would be particularly pertinent, given the multiple beneficial effects of GLP-1 on human metabolism and glucoregulation.[36] Notably, >50% of obese subjects with prediabetes treated with liraglutide (up to 3 mg/day) reverted to normal glucose status at 2 years; this was associated with ~8-kg weight loss from pretreatment baseline.[37] Besides normalizing glucose tolerance in >50% of subjects with prediabetes, liraglutide 3-mg treatment also markedly decreased the occurrence of prediabetes at 56 weeks among people who initially were normoglycemic (7.2% in liraglutide group vs. 20.7% in placebo group).[38]

For patients likely to be exposed to prolonged periods of diabetogenic and obesogenic regimens, randomized controlled trials to test the efficacy, safety, and cost-effectiveness of prophylactic treatment with antiobesity drugs (e.g., locaserin, phentermine/topiramate, bupropion/naltrexone, and liraglutide 3 mg) would be informative.

With regard to patient selection, appropriate candidates for diabetes pharmacoprophylactic trials could include high-risk patients awaiting organ transplantation; patients about to receive high-dose steroid therapy for inflammatory, rheumatological, or other conditions; and patients receiving highly active antiretroviral therapy[39,40] or antipsychotic agents,[41,42] who manifest early signs of metabolic decompensation. Other categories of patients may conceivably be added to the foregoing list. The benefits of prescribing any of the aforementioned medications to prevent drug-induced diabetes must be weighed against their potential adverse effects. The latter include gastrointestinal disturbances (metformin, acarbose, orlistat, GLP-1 receptor agonists; lorcaserin phentermine/topiramate, naltrexone/bupropion); warning regarding pancreatitis (GLP-1 receptor agonists, DPP-4 inhibitors); special precautions in people with renal dysfunction (metformin, DPP-4 inhibitors, GLP-1 receptor agonists, SGLT2 inhibitors); ketoacidosis (SGLT2 inhibitors); increased heart rate (GLP-1 receptor agonists); and multiple drug interactions, potential hypertensive crisis, neuropsychiatric reactions (lorcaserin phentermine/ topiramate, naltrexone/bupropion), among others.[43,44]

CONCLUSION

The prospect of selective use of medication to thwart a predictable outcome of drug-induced diabetes in a precise fashion currently is an elusive concept. There are numerous unknown elements to inform a rational approach to patient selection, prophylactic drug selection, timing and duration of intervention, determination of endpoints, and appropriate monitoring for adverse events. Furthermore, although metformin has been determined to be cost-effective and potentially cost-saving when used for preventing diabetes,[45,46] similar economic analyses have yet to be performed with regard to the cost-effectiveness of the other, more expensive medication options for diabetes prevention. By contrast, lifestyle intervention focusing on dietary and physical activity modifications are of proven efficacy and cost-effectiveness in preventing diabetes in high-risk individuals.[46] Thus, the current focus should be on the adaptation and implementation of effective lifestyle counseling for individuals receiving or about to receive medications that could increase their risk for diabetes. When a compelling rationale for the adjunctive use of medications to prevent diabetes in the highest-risk people is developed, that rationale would be incorporated into standard practice.

REFERENCES

1. Indian Health Services. IHS guidelines for care of adults with prediabetes and/or the metabolic syndrome in clinical settings, 2008. Available from http://aianp.ucdenver.edu/sdpi/common/initiative/DP_Appendices/DPIAN6%20IHS%20Guidelines%20PreDiabetes%20Metsyn%20Sept%202008.pdf. Accessed 3 July 2015

2. DPP Research Group. Reduction in the incidence of type 2 diabetes with lifestyle intervention or metformin. *N Engl J Med* 2002;346:393–403

3. Tuomilehto J, Lindstrom J, Eriksson J, Valle T, Hamalainen H. Prevention of type 2 diabetes mellitus by changes in lifestyle among subjects with impaired glucose tolerance. *N Engl J Med* 2001;344:1343–1350

4. Menza M, Vreeland B, Minsky S, et al. Managing atypical antipsychotic-associated weight gain: 12-month data on a multimodal weight control program. *J Clin Psychiatry* 2004;65:471–477

5. Hoffmann VP, Ahl J, Meyers A, et al. Wellness intervention for patients with serious and persistent mental illness. *J Clin Psychiatry* 2005;66:1576–1579

6. Canary Health. Available from http://www.canaryhealth.com/

7. Centers for Disease Control and Prevention. Diabetes Prevention Recognition Program. www.cdc.gov/diabetes/prevention/recognition

8. American Medical Association; Centers for Disease Control and Prevention (CDC). Prevent Diabetes STAT (Screen/Test/Act Today). Available from http://www.ama-assn.org/sub/prevent-diabetes-stat/

9. Ackermann RT, Marrero DG. Adapting the Diabetes Prevention Program lifestyle intervention for delivery in the community: the YMCA model. *Diabetes Educ* 2007;33:69,74–75,77–78

10. Albright AL, Gregg EW. Preventing type 2 diabetes in communities across the U.S.: the National Diabetes Prevention Program. *Am J Prev Med* 2013;44(4 Suppl. 4):S346–S351

11. Hays LM, Finch EA, Saha C, Marrero DG, Ackermann RT. Effect of self-efficacy on weight loss: a psychosocial analysis of a community-based adaptation of the Diabetes Prevention Program lifestyle intervention. *Diabetes Spectr* 2014;27:270–275

12. Pan XR, Li GW, Hu YH, Wang JX, Yang WY, An ZX, et al. Effects of diet and exercise in preventing NIDDM in people with impaired glucose tolerance: the Da Qing IGT and Diabetes Study. *Diabetes Care* 1997;20:537–544

13. Ramachandran A, Snehalatha C, Mary S, Mukesh B, Bhaskar AD, Vijay V; Indian Diabetes Prevention Programme (IDPP). The Indian Diabetes Prevention Programme shows that lifestyle modification and metformin prevent type 2 diabetes in Asian Indian subjects with impaired glucose tolerance (IDPP-1). *Diabetologia* 2006;49:289–297

14. Chiasson JL, Josse RG, Gomis R, Hanefeld M, Karasik A, Laakso M. STOP-NIDDM Trial Research Group. Acarbose for prevention of type 2 diabetes mellitus: the STOP-NIDDM randomised trial. *Lancet* 2002;359:2072–2077

15. Orgerson JS, Hauptman J, Boldrin MN, Sjöström L. XENical in the prevention of Diabetes in Obese Subjects (XENDOS) study: a randomized study of orlistat as an adjunct to lifestyle changes for the prevention of type 2 diabetes in obese patients. *Diabetes Care* 2004;27:155–161

16. Xiang AH, Peters RK, Kjos SL, Marroquin A, Goico J, Ochoa C, et al. Effects of pioglitazone on pancreatic β-cell function and diabetes risk in Hispanic women with prior gestational diabetes. *Diabetes* 2006;55:517–522

17. DREAM (Diabetes Reduction Assessment with Ramipril and Rosiglitazone Medication) Trial Investigators. Effect of rosiglitazone on the frequency of diabetes in patients with impaired glucose tolerance or impaired fasting glucose: a randomised controlled trial. *Lancet* 2006;368:1096–1105

18. DeFronzo RA, Tripathy D, Schwenke DC, Banerji M, Bray GA, Buchanan TA, Clement SC, Henry RR, Hodis HN, Kitabchi AE, Mack WJ, Mudaliar S, Ratner RE, Williams K, Stentz FB, Musi N, Reaven PD; ACT NOW Study. Pioglitazone for diabetes prevention in impaired glucose tolerance [published correction appears in *N Engl J Med* 2011;365:189]. *N Engl J Med* 2011;364:1104–1115

19. Zinman B, Harris SB, Neuman J, Gerstein HC, Retnakaran RR, Raboud J, Qi Y, Hanley AJ. Low-dose combination therapy with rosiglitazone and metformin to prevent type 2 diabetes mellitus (CANOE trial): a double-blind randomised controlled study. *Lancet* 2010;376:103–111

20a. NAVIGATOR Study Group. Effect of valsartan on the incidence of diabetes and cardiovascular events [published correction appears in *N Engl J Med* 2010;362:1748]. *N Engl J Med* 2010;362:1477–1490.

20b. NAVIGATOR Study Group. Effect of nateglinide on the incidence of diabetes and cardiovascular events. *N Engl J Med* 2010;362:1463–1476

21. DPP Research Group. Effects of withdrawal from metformin on the development of diabetes in the Diabetes Prevention Program. *Diabetes Care* 2003;26:977–980

22. DREAM Trial Investigators. Incidence of diabetes following ramipril or rosiglitazone withdrawal. *Diabetes Care* 2011;34:1265–1269

23. Ramachandran A, Snehalatha C, Mary S, Selvam S, Kumar CK, Seeli AC, Shetty AS. Pioglitazone does not enhance the effectiveness of lifestyle modification in preventing conversion of impaired glucose tolerance to diabetes in Asian Indians: results of the Indian Diabetes Prevention Programme-2 (IDPP-2). *Diabetologia* 2009;52:1019–1026

24. Echouffo-Tcheugui JB, Dagogo-Jack S. Preventing diabetes mellitus in developing countries. *Nat Rev Endocrinol* 2012;8:557–562

25. Greenway FL. Physiological adaptations to weight loss and factors favouring weight regain. *Int J Obes.* 21 Apr 2015. doi: 10.1038/ijo.2015.59 [Epub ahead of print]

26. Edeoga C, Dagogo-Jack S. Understanding and identifying pre-diabetes—can we halt the disease? *US Endocrinology* 2008;4:20–23

27. Akinci E, Banga A, Greder LV, Dutton JR, Slack JM. Reprogramming of pancreatic exocrine cells towards a β-cell character using Pdx1, Ngn3 and MafA. *Biochem J* 2012;442:539–550

28. Nathan DM, Davidson MB, DeFronzo RA, Heine RJ, Henry RR, Pratley R, Zinman B. Impaired fasting glucose and impaired glucose tolerance. *Diabetes Care* 2007;30:753–759

29. American Diabetes Association. Prevention or delay of type 2 diabetes. *Diabetes Care* 2015;38(Suppl. 1):S31–S32

30. Twigg SM, Kamp MC, Davis TM, Neylon EK, Flack JR; Australian Diabetes Society and Australian Diabetes Educators Association. Prediabetes: a position statement from the Australian Diabetes Society and Australian Diabetes Educators Association. *Med J Aust* 2007;186:461–465

31. Dagogo-Jack S, Askari H, Tykodi G. Glucoregulatory physiology in subjects with low-normal, high-normal, or impaired fasting glucose. *J Clin Endocrinol Metab* 2009;94:2031–2036

32. Kanat M, Mari A, Norton L, Winnier D, DeFronzo RA, Jenkinson C, Abdul-Ghani MA. Distinct β-cell defects in impaired fasting glucose and impaired glucose tolerance. *Diabetes* 2012;61:447–453

33. Rhee MK, Herrick K, Ziemer DC, Vaccarino V, Weintraub WS, Narayan KM, et al. Many Americans have pre-diabetes and should be considered for metformin therapy. *Diabetes Care* 2010;33:49–54

34. DPP Research Group. Long-term safety, tolerability, and weight loss associated with metformin in the Diabetes Prevention Program Outcomes Study. *Diabetes Care* 2012;35:731–737

35. Garber AJ, Blonde L, Bloomgarden JT, Dagogo-Jack S. Bromocriptine-QR for type 2 diabetes: AACE Expert Panel review of its potential place in therapy. *Endocr Pract* 2013;19:100–106

36. Drucker DJ, Sherman SI, Bergenstal RM, Buse JB. The safety of incretin-based therapies—review of the scientific evidence. *J Clin Endocrinol Metab* 2011;96:2027–2031

37. Astrup A, Carraro R, Finer N, Harper A, Kunesova M, Lean MEJ, et al. Safety, tolerability and sustained weight loss over 2 years with the once-daily human GLP-1 analog, liraglutide. *Int J Obes* (Lond) 2012;36:843–854

38. Pi-Sunyer X, Astrup A, Fujioka K, et al. A randomized, controlled trial of 3.0 mg of liraglutide in weight management. *N Engl J Med* 2015;373:11–22

39. Hadigan C, Corcoran C, Basgoz N, Davis B, Sax P, Grinspoon S. Metformin in the treatment of HIV lipodystrophy syndrome: a randomized controlled trial. *JAMA* 2000;284:472–427

40. Goodwin SR, Reeds DN, Royal M, Struthers H, Laciny E, Yarasheski, KE. Dipeptidyl peptidase IV inhibition does not adversely affect immune or virological status in HIV infected men and women: a pilot safety study. *J Clin Endocrinol Metab* 2013; 98:743–751

41. Khan AY, Macaluso M, McHale RJ, Dahmen MM, Girrens K, Ali F. The adjunctive use of metformin to treat or prevent atypical antipsychotic-induced weight gain: a review. *J Psychiatr Pract* 2010;16:289–296

42. Ellinger LK, Ipema HJ, Stachnik JM. Efficacy of metformin and topiramate in prevention and treatment of second-generation antipsychotic-induced weight gain. *Ann Pharmacother* 2010;44:668–679

43. Citrome L. Editorial. Lorcaserin, phentermine topiramate combination, and naltrexone bupropion combination for weight loss: the 15-min challenge to sort these agents out. *Int J Clin Pract* 2014;68:1401–1405.

44. Peters AL, Buschur EO, Buse JB, Cohan P, Diner JC, Hirsch IB. Euglycemic diabetic ketoacidosis: a potential complication of treatment with sodium-glucose cotransporter 2 inhibition. *Diabetes Care* 2015;38:1687–1693

45. Ramachandran A, Snehalatha C, Yamuna A, Mary S, Ping Z. Cost-effectiveness of the interventions in the primary prevention of diabetes among Asian Indians: within-trial results of the Indian Diabetes Prevention Programme (IDPP). *Diabetes Care* 2007;30:2548–2552

46. Herman WH, Edelstein SL, Ratner RE, et al., Diabetes Prevention Program Research Group. The 10-year cost-effectiveness of lifestyle intervention or metformin for diabetes prevention: an intent-to-treat analysis of the DPP/DPPOS. *Diabetes Care* 2012;35:723–730

Index

Note: page numbers followed by *f* refer to figures. Page numbers followed by *t* refer to tables.

A

A1c. *See* hemoglobin A1c
α-adrenergic receptor, 89
α-adrenoreceptor blocker, 48
α-andrenergic blocker, 107
abacavir, 71*t*
acarbose, 110, 114
ACE inhibitor. *See* angiotensin-converting enzyme (ACE) inhibitor
α-cell, 8–9
acetaminophen, 97–98
acetoacetate, 89
acetyl CoA carboxylase (ACC), 7
acetyl-coenzyme A (acetyl CoA), 6*f*, 7, 89
acromegaly, 99
Actos Now for the Prevention of Diabetes (ACT NOW), 110*t*, 111
adenosine triphosphate (ATP)–sensitive potassium channel (KATP), 8
adenylate cyclase, 89
adipocyte, 7, 24
adiponectin, 7, 97
adiponectin gene, 87
adipose tissue, 89
African American population, 5
age, 4
α-glucosidase inhibitor, 27, 70
α-Interferon, 15*t*
Akt/protein kinase B (PKB), 6

alcohol/alcoholism, 17–18, 85
alcoholic pancreatitis, 85
aldosterone, 24
allograft, 26–27
alloxan, 17
Ambrose, PG, 68
American Association of Clinical Endocrinologists (AACE), 101
American Cancer Society (ACS), 40
American Diabetes Association (ADA), 1, 2*f*, 85, 100–102, 112
American Diabetes Association Consensus Panel, 77
American Heart Association (AHA), 40
American Medical Association (AMA), 109
American Urological Association (AUA), 40
amphetamine, 89–90
amprenavir, 69
amputation, 62
anabolic steroid, 39
anakinra, 28
androgen, 36–38
androgen-deprivation therapy (ADT), 40
angiogenesis, 62
angiotensin-converting enzyme (ACE) inhibitor, 47–49, 107
angiotensin receptor blocker (ARBs), 48–49, 107
Anglo- Scandinavian Cardiac Outcomes Trial (ASCOT), 47

methylenedioxy-methamphetamine (MDMA or Ecstasy), 89–90
methylxanthine, 55
metoprolol, 48
metreleptin, 71
Mexican American population, 5
microalbuminuria, 49, 62
microvascular complication, 57, 62
mineralocorticoid, 24
minoxidil, 50
mitochondrial dysfunction, 69
monitoring, 77
monogenic syndrome, 2
monozygotic (identical) twins, 3
moxifloxacin, 68
myocardial infarction, 47, 58
myocyte, 7

N

naloxone, 87–89
naltrexone, 88
National Health and Nutrition Examination Survey (NHANES), 4–5, 86
National Health and Nutrition Examination Survey (NHANES) III, 86
National Institutes of Health (NIH), 4, 75
NAVIGATOR trial, 48, 110*t*, 111
nelfinavir, 69
neogenesis, 112
nephropathy, 26
neuropathic pain, 99
neuropathy, 49, 62, 85, 88–89
neuropsychiatric reaction, 115
neurosurgery, 99
nevirapine, 71
new-onset diabetes, 48, 49*f*, 86
new-onset diabetes after transplantation (NODAT), 25–27
niacin, 58

NICE-SUGAR (Normoglycemia in Intensive Care Evaluation-Survival Using Glucose Algorithm Regulation) study, 101
nicotinamide, 17
nicotine, 86
nicotinic acid, 15*t*, 57–58, 107
nitric oxide synthase, 62
nondiabetic ketoacidosis, 99
nonesterified fatty acids (NEFAs), 7, 55, 57, 89
non-Hispanic black population, 5
non-Hispanic white population, 5
nonketotic hyperosmolar syndrome, 89
non-nucleoside RT inhibitor, 71*t*
nonsteroidal anti-inflammatory drugs (NSAIDs), 15*t*, 97–98
norepinephrine, 89–90
norepinephrine reuptake inhibitors, 79
ntiretroviral agents, 71
nucleoside analog, 69–70, 71*t*
nucleoside RT inhibitor, 71*t*
nutrient flux, 15*t*

O

obesity, 67, 86, 88
obesogenic regimen, 114
olanzapine, 75–76
opioid, 87–89
opioid-associated obesity, 88
oral antidiabetic medication, 71
oral contraceptive (OC), 35–36
oral contraceptive-induced diabetes, 36
oral glucose tolerance test (OGTT), 1, 2*f*, 26, 35–36, 113
oral medication, 55
organic cation transporter 1 (OCT1), 17
organ transplantation, 24–25, 114
orlistat, 110, 110*t*, 114